Biometry
Technology, Trends and Applications

Editors

Ricardo A. Ramirez-Mendoza
Jorge de J. Lozoya-Santos
Ricardo Zavala-Yoé
Luz María Alonso-Valerdi
Ruben Morales-Menendez
Belinda Carrión
Pedro Ponce Cruz
Hugo G. Gonzalez-Hernandez
Tecnologico de Monterrey
School of Engineering and Sciences
Monterrey, Mexico

CRC Press
Taylor & Francis Group
Boca Raton London New York

CRC Press is an imprint of the
Taylor & Francis Group, an **informa** business

A SCIENCE PUBLISHERS BOOK

First edition published 2022
by CRC Press
6000 Broken Sound Parkway NW, Suite 300, Boca Raton, FL 33487-2742

and by CRC Press
4 Park Square, Milton Park, Abingdon, Oxon OX14 4RN

© 2022 Taylor & Francis Group, LLC

CRC Press is an imprint of Taylor & Francis Group, an Informa business

Library of Congress Cataloging-in-Publication Data (applied for)

ISBN: 978-0-367-70247-2 (hbk)
ISBN: 978-0-367-70250-2 (pbk)
ISBN: 978-1-003-14524-0 (ebk)

DOI: 10.1201/9781003145240

Typeset in Times New Roman
by Radiant Productions

Preface

Throughout history, humankind has been progressing steadily in the generation of knowledge and applications using such findings. In this context, different revolutions have emerged across the years, such as in agriculture, industry, technology, science, and, most recently, information. Information technologies refer to the analysis, structuring and interpretation of vast amounts of data and information available as an endless resource for research, and development in different fields. Healthcare represents one among many other fields with increasing applications of information technologies.

Biometric systems are some of the most notorious representatives of this type of technology. These systems obtain relevant information regarding our bodies and behaviors. Many innovative solutions under this scheme generate biosensors, the development of personalized healthcare services, intelligent fitness applications, wearable devices, and algorithms for predicting pathologies and health risks based on readings and analyses of physiological features, among other data. Thus, biometric systems provide the means to identify, authenticate, and model individuals in a reliable way through unique physiological and behavioral features. Ultimately, such systems generate information and knowledge about the health and behavior of humans.

Biometrics has been an essential component in security, military, and criminology, and new types of biometric systems are emerging as essential platforms in healthcare, smart cities, and industrial business. Former and seminal applications in health, ergonomics, transportation, industry, education, neuromarketing, and arts could lead these efforts to develop biometric systems to become an everyday asset. Such systems will strongly support the health, wellness, and performance of humans. These are current opportunities as the reliability and wearability of these technologies dare and inspire our researchers to look for innovative solutions for humanity.

This book presents a compilation of biometric technologies studied and developed in various research groups in Tecnologico de Monterrey, Mexico. A summary of biometric systems as a whole provides a starting point for all readers. It explains the principles behind physiological and behavioral biometrics. It explores different types of commercial and experimental technology and current and future applications in the fields of security, military, criminology, healthcare, education, business, and marketing.

The following chapters include more in-depth descriptions of research methods and results from studies where biometric systems are the main protagonists. Among the selected topics are

- The analysis of brain signals, or electroencephalography (EEG) in mobile and home EEG in natural environments of children, as well as in the monitoring of epileptic encephalopathies in children.
- The development of functional Human Machine Interfaces (HMI) and Brain-Computer Interfaces (BCI).
- A description of the BCI framework and novel applications-oriented towards rehabilitation, human performance, and treatment monitoring.
- Some techniques as machine learning, deep learning, and artificial intelligence aid in the diagnosis, seizure detection, and data-centered medical decisions.

Finally, the authors highlight that this book is a compilation of biometric systems, and many other exciting research proposals exist. Therefore, we hope readers will become interested in such technology, and the invitation is open to keep researching and innovating in this field.

November 22nd, 2021

Ricardo A. Ramirez-Mendoza
Monterrey, Mexico

To Thelma, Jehosefat, Jorge, Ignacio, Victoria and Georgina,
We are one. — **J. Lozoya-Santos**

To Pily, Montse, Georgy, Marianne, my parents
and my grandparents. — **R. Morales-Menéndez**

To my very dear little daughter Arantza,
for her love and strength. — **R. Zavala-Yoé**

To future biomedical engineers and scientists where technology
and health knowledge can meet to provide better
health care. — **B. Carrión**

To my family and friends that reminded of enjoying the little
detours in life. — **E.A. Martínez-Ríos**

To my parents Gandhi and Isabel, my sister Guadalupe
and my dear Vic for their love and support. — **J.I. Méndez**

To my beloved wife Saracelly and my daughter Regina,
for their support and loving patience. — **H.G. Gonzalez-Hernandez**

To my wife Lolis and my children
Andrea, Ilse and Diego. — **D. Antonio-Torres**

For my family, my haven of endless
motivation. — **W. Carballo-Hernandez**

To Pedro and Jamie, my children who teach me every day
my life how to be happy. — **P. Ponce Cruz**

The work dignifies, the discipline magnifies and the
constancy exalts. — **L.M. Alonso-Valerdi**

My deepest thanks to God for allowing me to finish
this book. — **R.A. Ramirez-Mendoza**

Contents

5. Mobile and Home Electroencephalography in the Usual Environment of Children   97

Belinda Carrion and *Luis Felipe Herrera Padilla*

6. Health: Human-Machine Interaction, Medical Robotics, Patient Rehabilitation   110

Pedro Ponce, Erick Axel Martínez-Ríos, Juana Isabel Méndez, Arturo Molina and *Ricardo A Ramirez-Mendoza*

Symbol Description

2D-DWT	Two Dimensional Discrete Wavelet Transform	CZP	Clonazepam
ACD	Asthma Control Diary	CZP	Clorasepate dipotassium
ADC	Analog to Digital Converter	DAC	Digital to Analog Converter
AED	Antiepileptic Drugs	DBMSE	Dynamic Bivariate Multiscale Entropy
AI	Artificial Intelligence	DBP	Digital Biosignal Processing
AL	Axial Length		
AMFC	Adaptive Margin Fisher's Criterion	DBSCAN	Density-Based Spatial Clustering of Applications with Noise
ANN	Artificial Neural Networks		
APSoC	All-programmable System-On-Chip	DHPLC	Denaturing High-Performance Liquid Chromatography
ASD	Autism Spectrum Disorder		
ATX	Atomoxetine	DNA	Deoxyribonucleic acid
BaaS	Biometrics as a Service	DNN	Deep Neural Network
BCG	Ballistocardiography	DPN	Diabetic Poly Neuropathy
BCI	Brain Computer Interface	DTI	Diffusion Tensor Imaging
BMSE	Bivariate Multiscale Entropy	ECG	Electrocardiography
		ECGi	Electrocardiographic Imaging
BOD	Biochemical Oxygen Demand		
		ECoG	Electrocorticography
BOLD	Blood Oxygen Level Dependent	EDA	Electrodermal Activity
		EEG	Electroencephalogram
BP	Blood Pressure	EMG	Electromyography
CE	Capillary Electrophoresis	EMU	Epylepsy Monitoring Units
CHB-MIT	Child Hospital Boston-MIT		
		EOG	Electrooculography
CLB	Clobazam	ERD	Event-Related Desynchronization
CMR	Cardiac Magnetic Resonance		
		ER-HR	Event-Related Heart Rate
CNN	Convolutional Neural Network	ERP	Event-Related Potential
		ERS	Event-Related Synchronization
CNS	Central Nervous System		
CV	Cross Validation	ESM	Ethosuximide
CWT	Continuous Wavelet Transform	EW	Electric Wheelchair
		FCG	Fonocardiogram

FLC	Fuzzy Logic Controllers	LDA	Linear Discriminant
FNIRS	Functional Near Infrarred		Analysis
	Spectroscopy	LEV	Levetiracetam
FPGA	Field-Programmable Gate	LTG	Lamotrigina
	Array	MCG	Magnetocardiography
FRS	Force Resistive Sensor	MDZ	Midazolam
GIN	Genetic Identification	MEG	Magnetoencephalography
	Number	MFCC	Mel-Frequency Cepstral
GLPF	Gaussian Low-Pass Filter		Coefficients
GMM	Gaussian Mixture Model	MIT	Massachusetts Institute of
GPS	Global Positioning System		Technology
GSR	Galvanic Skin Response	MK-BOP	Multi Kernelled Bijection
GUI	Graphical User Interface		Octal Pattern
HAR	Human Activity	ML	Machine Learning
	Recognition	MMC	Maximum Margin
HCI	Human Computer		Criterion
	Interaction	MMRGlu	Myocardium Metabolic
HE	Histogram equalization		Rate for Glucose
HFCC	Human-Factor Cepstral	MRI	Magnetic Resonance
	Coefficients		Imaging
HIBS	Human Identification	MSE	Multiscale Entropy
	Barcode System	NCA	Neighbor Component
HMI	Human Machine Interface		Analysis
HMM	Hidden Markov Model	NCS	Nerve Conduction Study
HOG	Histogram of Oriented	NM	Neuro-Marketing
	Gradient	ORA	Optiwave Refractive
HR	Heart Rate		Analysis
HRV	Heart Rate Variability	OSA	Obstructive Sleep Apnea
ICA	Independent Component	OSAS	Obstructive Sleep Apnea
	Analysis		Syndrome
ID	Identity	PA	Piracetam
IHC	Inner Hair Cell Coefficient	PB	Phenobarbital
IIR	Infinite Impulse Response	PCA	Principal Component
IMI	Imipramine		Analysis
IoBT	Internet of Biometric	PCR	Polymerase Chain
	Things		Reaction
IoT	Internet of Things	PED	Performance Enhancing
IRF	Iterative ReliefF		Drugs
ISCEV	International Society for	PET	Positron Emission
	Clinical Electrophysiology		Tomography
	of Vision	PG	PolyGraphy
kNN	k-Nearest Neighbors	PNS	Peripheral Nervous
LCM	Lacosamide		System
		PPG	Photoplethysmography

PRM	Primidone
PSE	Prednisone
PSG	Polysomnography
PSO	Particle Swarm Optimization
PVE	Partial Volume Effect
RAM	Random-access memory
RBF	Radial Basis Function
RFID	Radio Frequency Identification
RGB	Red-Green-Blue
RNN	Recurrent Neural Network
RS	Robin Sequence
RSP	Respiration
SBB	Social Behavioral Biometrics
SC	Skin conductance
SCC	Stress Classification Coefficient
SER	Speech Emotion Recognition
SG	Serious Games
SGA	Simple Genetic Algorithm
SKT	Skin Temperature
SLM	Supervised Learning Methods
SNP	Single-Nucleotide Polymorphism
SRC	Sparse Representation Classifier
STEM	Science, Technology, Engineering, and Mathematics
STR	Short Tandem Repeat
SSS	Small Sample Size
SURF	Speeded-Up Robust Features
SVD	Singular Value Decomposition
SVM	Support Vector Machine
T2D	Type 2 Diabetes
TD	Typically Developed
TEG	Thermoelectric generator
TFB	Triangular Filter Bank
TFBCC	Triangular Filter Bank Cepstral Coefficients
TLE	Temporal Lobe Epilepsy
TP	Ternary Pattern
TPM	Topiramate
TRD	Treatment-Resistant Depression
TV	Television
UCD	User-Centered Design
ULM	Unsupervised Learning Methods
UL-OCT	Ultra-Long scan depth Optical Coherence Tomography
UMRT	Unique Mapped Real Transform
UV	Ultraviolet
VPA	Valproate Sodium
VPA+	Magnesium Valproate
VT	Ventricular Tachycardia
WDD	Wrist-Worn Device
XLH	X-Linked Hypophosphatemia
ZNS	Zonisamide
dpt	Dioptre (optical power of a lens)
i	Index
f	Fundamental frequency of the biosignal oscillation
k	Number of groups, clusters, etc.
l	Lower
mHealth	Mobile health
mph	Miles per hour
n	Number of records
s	Scaling factor
u	Upper
CA	Class Attribute
D	Dataset
E	Entropy
Hz	Hertz
P	Probability

1

Current and Future Biometrics: Technology and Applications

Jorge de J Lozoya-Santos,* Mauricio A Ramírez-Moreno, Gladys G Diaz-Armas, Luis F Acosta-Soto, Milton O Candela Leal, Rafael Abrego-Ramos and *Ricardo A Ramirez-Mendoza*

1.1 Introduction

This chapter will explore biometric definitions, types, commercial and experimental technology as well as current and potential applications. Biometrics considers the means of identifying, authenticating and modeling individuals in a reliable way through the use of unique physiological and behavioral characteristics. The current methods, apparatus and techniques are summarized for each biometric physical body measure (physiological) to gait (behavioral) passing by finger print and facial recognition, speech and human-machine interactions. Biometrics has been an important component in different applications such as security, military aspects and criminology. Biometric systems appear to be mandatory in some applications becoming an essential in healthcare, smart cities and industrial businesses. Some seminal applications in education, neuromarketing and arts could lead all the efforts for biometrics to become an every day asset for the increasing concern for health and human performances in the future world.

1.2 Biometrics

Biometrics is the discipline and techniques involving the recognition, modeling and understanding of the individuals based on their distinctive behavioral, physiological and cognitive characteristics, rather than using something known or possessed, [281, 172].

The utilized techniques in biometrics cover data acquisition, data analysis and characterization, theoretical - heuristic modeling, computational simulation and visualization techniques, [140, 539, 212]. Classical applications have been focused on

School of Engineering and Sciences, Tecnologico de Monterrey, Monterrey, Mexico.

* Corresponding author: jorge.lozoya@tec.mx

agriculture, [87], environmental science, biology, [521, 492], and medical sciences, [393].

A biometric system is a pattern recognition system that establishes the authenticity of a specific physiological or behavioral characteristic possessed by a user, [385]. However, digital transformation pushes biometric systems as data acquisition systems with application to the description, prediction, and imitation of human behavior for several purposes as personalization of services and remote body monitoring [308, 65]. Typically, a biometric system is used for: (a) Logical Access Control; (b) Physical Access Control; (c) Time and Attendance; (d) Law Enforcement; and (e) Surveillance. Novel applications are consumer behavior [539], sports [42], and workforce wellness [98, 441].

The fields of biometric applications are product differentiators, and, forensic and government services. Mainly the goal of these systems is user/person identification, [530]. Several biometric traits can be used, [445]. Biometric Commercial applications focus on authenticating users to give them some kind of privilege or access, [574].

1.2.1 Physiological biometrics

Physiological biometrics refer to physical measurements of the human body and thus they vary from person to person, [269]. Most of the times it is necessary to use a specialized sensor/hardware to perform the data acquisition, and its likelihood for reliable human identification is very high, [149]. A non exhaustive list of research results evidences the scientific community interest in these biometrics: ear, [396], electroencephalgraph, [357], face, [301], face thermography, [215], fingerprint, [82], [251], hand geometry, [266], iris, [325], and wrist vein, [421], Figure 1.1. A region-based classification, [530], consists of: (a) hand region; (b) facial region; (c) ocular region; and (d) medico-chemical phenomena, Figure 1.1. In Table 1.1, there are some examples of the most used physiological biometrics and how well they perform comparing different requirements, [149].

TABLE 1.1: Physiological biometrics, [149].

Characteristic	Universality	Distinctiveness	Collectabillity	Performance	Acceptability
Ear	Medium	Medium	Medium	Medium	High
Hand Geometry	Medium	Medium	High	Medium	Medium
Fingerprint	Medium	High	Medium	High	Medium
Face	High	Low	High	Low	High
Iris	High	High	Medium	High	Low
Voice	Medium	Low	Medium	Low	High

1.2.2 Behavioral biometrics

Behavioral biometrics are the behavioral characteristics that relate to the pattern of people doing something (authorship, body dynamics, performance and dynamics of

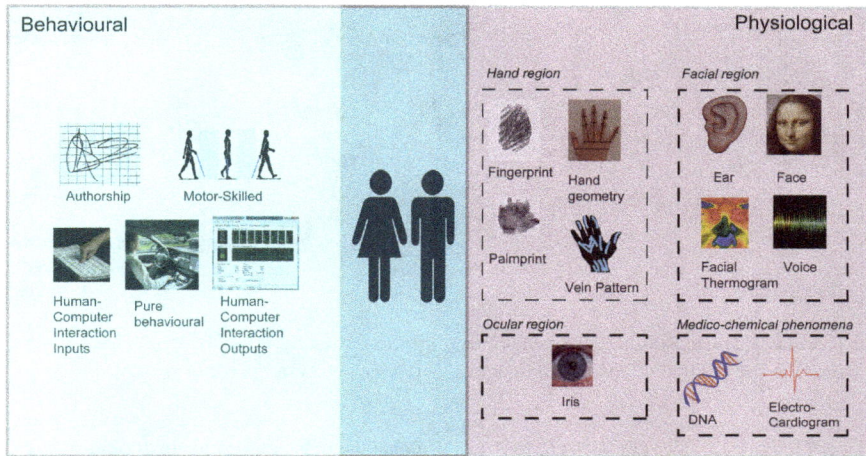

FIGURE 1.1: Main biometric traits, [281], [530], [574], [232]. In the biometric literature, these characteristics are referred to as traits, indicators, identifiers.

things operated/used by humans), [574], [269], Figure 1.1. Behavioral biometrics have advantages over physiological biometric technologies. They can be collected non-obtrusively, often do not require any special hardware and they are very cost effective. Most of the behavioural biometrics have been shown to provide sufficiently high accuracy identity verification, [574], although performance is generally lower than with physiological biometrics, [381]. Extensive research efforts during the years gone by have shown this topic as an open issue with opportunities and challenges: behaviour profile, [23], driving style, [442], [106], gait, [66], [107], handwriting, [43], human computer interaction, [146], keystroke dynamics [202], [168], mouse dynamics, [14], network traffic, [21], social network interaction, [507], walking sound, [67], and wearable dynamics, [17].

Five categories have been proposed in [574]: (a) authorship-based (signature, text, drawing, painting), (b) Human Computer Interaction (*HCI*)-based (keystroke, mouse, change of software screens), (c) *HCI*-Performance-based (network traffic, registry access, storage activity), (d) motor-skill based (gait, handwriting), and (e) pure behavioural (performance analysis of how an individual operates a thing).

Human Activity Recognition (*HAR*) provides accurate and opportune information on activities and behaviors of persons [286]. It uses behavioral biometrics. The recognition of human activities is key for several fields like medical, military, and security applications. However, recognizing activities requires specificity according to the field of application to provide useful feedback to the generated information end user. The *HAR* can be divided in those activities performed by a person in spaces or using devices or systems, Figure 1.2.

Using the human activity classification using devices or systems, a set of behavioural biometrics that can be acquired when using mobile devices, non-mobile devices with embedded computer (personal computer or systems such as TV or in-

Rowing, lifting weights, spinning, nordic walking, doing push ups.		Chewing, speaking, swallowing, sighing, moving the head.		**Human activity using spaces**
Exercise/ fitness		**Upper body**		
Walking, running, sitting, standing still, lying, climbing stairs, descending stairs	Crawling, kneeling, situation assessment, *opening a door.*	Eating, drinking, reading, *brushing teeth,* stretching, scrubbing, vacuuming	Riding a bus	
Ambulation	**Military**	**Daily activities**	**Transportation**	**HAR**
Riding escalator Riding elevator.		Phone usage, working at the PC, watching TV.	Cycling Driving.	**Human activity using devices or systems**

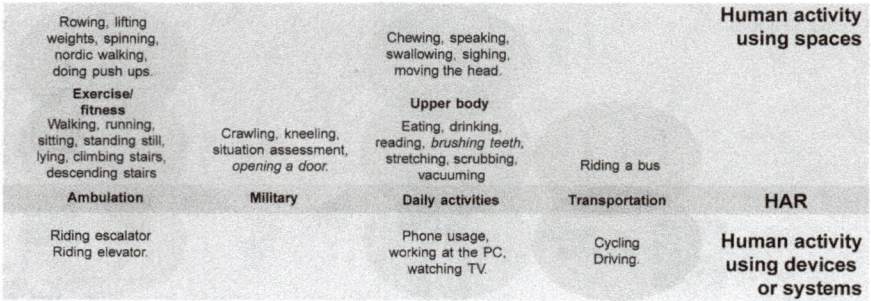

FIGURE 1.2: Classification of behavioural biometrics using the *HAR* from [286] (italic bold words) in the context of the use of spaces and devices or systems (bold words).

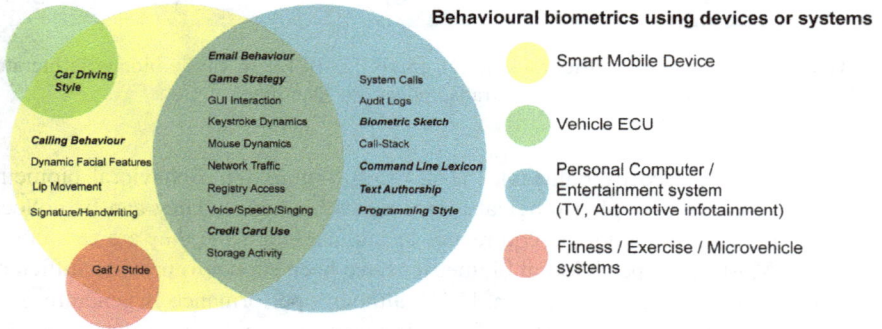

Behavioural biometrics using devices or systems

Car Driving Style

Email Behaviour
Game Strategy
GUI Interaction
Keystroke Dynamics
Mouse Dynamics
Network Traffic
Registry Access
Voice/Speech/Singing
Credit Card Use
Storage Activity

System Calls
Audit Logs
Biometric Sketch
Call-Stack
Command Line Lexicon
Text Authorship
Programming Style

Calling Behaviour
Dynamic Facial Features
Lip Movement
Signature/Handwriting

Gait / Stride

Smart Mobile Device

Vehicle ECU

Personal Computer / Entertainment system (TV, Automotive infotainment)

Fitness / Exercise / Microvehicle systems

FIGURE 1.3: Classification of behavioural biometrics using systems or devices according to the required hardware to be acquired and the purely behavioural property. Modified from, [308]. Bold words were classified in [574] as pure behavioural biometrics.

fotainment systems), microvehicles or fitness equipment and a vehicle. It shows that mobile and non-mobile devices, can deliver almost the same biometrics, Figure 1.3, and smart mobile devices (tablet, smartphone) and smart vehicles or microvehicles can deliver motor-skilled and performance-based biometrics. So, it is possible to get behavioural biometrics from everybody since the use of the Internet of Things technology in products and equipment is very common and continuous on a daily basis, [106].

A taxonomy to classify the biometrics from a sensorial point of view proposes a classification based on human senses: hearing, sight, smell, touch and metadata, [381]. This classification approach can be used for that presented in Figures 1.1–1.3 since a human, when using at least one sense, identifying a person for both type of biometrics, physiological or behavioural, depends on their availability. A summary of all behavioural biometrics where the human activity classifies those based on the creation of expression, device or system use and space use links the *HAR* application, Figure 1.4.

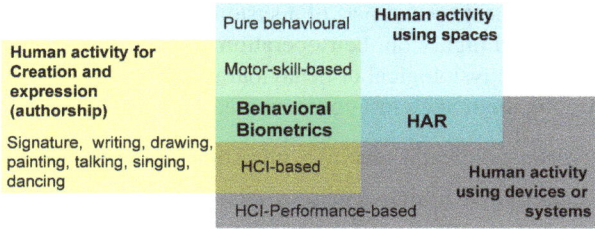

FIGURE 1.4: Behavioural biometrics.

1.3 Technology

This section breaks down the technology of biometric systems: sensors, methods, and the typical setup. Commercial technology presents the available devices and equipment for enabling biometric applications.

1.3.1 Sensors

A biometric system is composed of four parts [126, 233]: (a) a *sensor module* to obtain the biometric data, (b) a *feature extraction module* to select the information of interest, (c) a *matching and decision-making module* that decides if the user's identity is accepted based on the stored information, and (d) a *system database* acting as a repository for the biometric information of the authorized users, Figure 1.5.

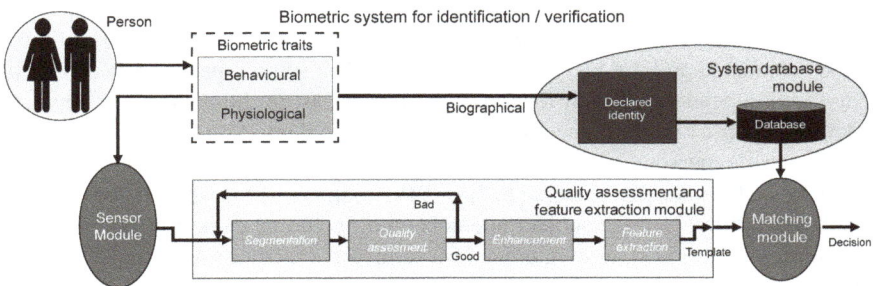

FIGURE 1.5: Biometric system.

For a biometric system to be reliable, it needs to fulfill certain parameters, including the acceptance of the public (people should be willing to use it), the use of a unique and time-invariant individual characteristic, and the possibility for acquisition and digitization of the human trait without inconvenience to the individual. It is also very important that the chosen characteristic is shown by the whole population that is expected to use the system [233, 533].

Sensors are the most crucial part of a system, as the performance indexes of the whole system depend highly on their operation and correct use [395, 411]. For this reason, all features (physiological or behavioural) can be obtained by different types of sensors. Among them, the most common are:

1. Fingerprints: optical, capacitive, ultrasonic or thermal sensors [10, 425].
2. Voice: capacitive or magnetic sensors (microphones) [262].
3. Vein recognition: infrared optical sensors, depending on the site of analysis (retina, finger, hand) [425, 422].
4. Gait: capacitive sensors (accelerometers) [177].
5. Iris: optical sensors with infrared illumination (cameras) [425, 57].
6. Face: optical or thermal sensors [425, 57].
7. Signature: optical and movement sensors [159].

Most biometric identifiers are acquired as an image, except for voice recognition or chemical-based signals (e.g., odor, DNA) [233]. For this reason, the resolution of the camera will affect the quality of the authentication, leading to possible errors. According to [411], these errors can be classified as *Failure to Enroll, False Match, False Non-Match, False Negative Identification and False Positive Identification.*

In all sensor types, the correct interaction between the user and the system is crucial to avoid these types of errors, especially, failure to enroll [233]. It is important to mention that, due to the changing nature of many traits, time can also affect the correct identification of the user [411].

1.3.2   Typical setups

For successful recognition, biometric systems must be set up according to the trait to be evaluated and the body part related to it. The setup types have been classified by [338] depending on their level of intrusiveness as: in-the-person, for implantable devices such as cardiac pacemakers or neural implants (e.g., the Neuralink chip) [117]; on-the-person, where devices are attached to the body, including any wearable sensor, such as accelerometers [177] or PPG systems [400]; and off-the-person, for hardware with which the subject interacts with, including cameras [245], keyboards, or microphones [578], among others. More invasive methods are usually focused on the acquisition of biosignals, and are useful to avoid complications that happen with non-invasive devices, such as distortions that avoid matching [533]. Nevertheless, less invasive methods are more acceptable to the public, are more suitable for large-scale applications and their use is cost-effective [177]. Finally, non-invasive methods can be embedded in existing systems, such as mobile phones, as they already have the necessary sensors and their discriminating power is enough to ensure high-level security [234].

These systems can also be classified as unimodal and multimodal, depending on the number of traits used to identify the user. Normally, a single feature is enough to distinguish between subjects, but when the chosen characteristic is time variant, e.g., fingerprints, or it lacks individuality, face recognition, it is useful to have a second attribute.

Multimodal systems were introduced to avoid problems related to the use of only one type of trait, improving the universality of the system and reducing the failure to enroll rate [376]. They contain the same parts as mentioned in the previous section, and they can use a fusion strategy to incorporate the information obtained from the set of sensors or consider each trait as an independent feature [376, 126]. In the present day, multimodal systems with different fusion levels are being developed as an alternative to improve the performance and usability of existing systems [376]. The appearance of novel multimodal systems is expected in the upcoming years.

1.3.3 Methods

Physiological recognition is one of the main research directions of biometrics, this category comprises biometrics based on images. One of the main difficulties that hinder this task is the large dimension of this data, as images are interpreted by a computer as a matrix of m x n dimensions composed of RGB values that range from 0 to 255, represented by the following image matrix X:

$$X_{m,n} = \begin{bmatrix} x_{1,1} & x_{1,2} & \cdots & x_{1,n} \\ x_{2,1} & x_{2,2} & \cdots & x_{2,n} \\ \vdots & \vdots & \ddots & \vdots \\ x_{m,1} & x_{m,2} & \cdots & x_{m,n} \end{bmatrix} \tag{1.1}$$

The matrix provided before is considered as high dimensional data, therefore a common approach for using the image is reducing its dimensions; researchers are prone to use algorithms to reduce the data dimensions and a popular option is the unsupervised algorithm PCA (Principal Component Analysis), which uses SVD (Singular Value Decomposition) to reduce the dimensions that the matrix has and transforms it into a low-dimensional subspace, whose vectors agree to the directions with maximal variances [575]. However, this statistical method ignores the class label and it does not suffice to identify to classify, for example, a human face, thus is combined with a non-linear classifier such as SVM (support vector machine) which locates an optimal hyper-plane to find the least Euclidean distance between the train image eigenvectors and the test image eigenvectors, and so the nearest distance is considered to be the same person. The concept is based on the classical face recognition algorithm knows as "Eigenface", proposed by the Massachusetts Institute of Technology (MIT) [528], and applies to many of the physiological recognition algorithms that use images in biometrics. In order to utilize a PCA + SVM algorithm, data has to first pass through a pre-processing stage by scaling, normalizing and applying image filters to reduce noise, furthermore, it is combined with an additional technique to improve accuracy, efficiency or other parameters of interest; among the recent techniques that had been used are: *(a)* Speeded-Up Robust Features (SURF) matching the source image with the database [468], *(b)* Histogram equalization (HE) and Guassian low-pass filter (GLPF) solving full illumination variation [297], *(c)* Simple Genetic Algorithm (SGA) optimizing the process of feature search [590], *(d)* Particle Swarm Optimization (PSO) implementing a feature selection [472], *(e)* Histogram of Oriented Gradient (HOG) matching features from the gallery with the probe [119], *(f)* Two Dimensional Discrete Wavelet Transform (2D-DWT) reducing computational complexity when using PCA [571].

Fingerprint recognition uses similar methods, as it applies image processing techniques to get a Thinned Fingerprint, such as: *(a)* Contrast stretching, *(b)* Gray-levels smoothing, *(c)* Histogram equalization, *(d)* Wiener filtering, then normalizes the data and extracts the features using ridge extracting [359]. After the pre-processing for fingerprint images aforementioned, a variety of machine learning methods including SVM, Recurrent Neural Networks (RNNs), K-means (clusters of k classes with the least Euclidean distances between each other) and even graph theory are applied to classify the distinct features, i.e., arch-type, a fingerprint has [560], and so match one fingerprint with another. In addition, a recent algorithm that uses generalized minutiae-neighbor based fingerprint encoding used a Field Programmable Gate array (FPGA) which employed Distributed RAM to match 2.75 million fingerprints per second while maintaining a low error rate [464]; this could subsequently provide efficient large-scale applications that massively match and authenticate.

There are in fact other dimensionality reduction techniques, another basic approach on contrasting and finding similarities across this high dimensional data is using Linear Discriminant Analysis (LDA), which has some similarities with PCA, although it keeps the class and so the algorithm in question is then a supervised batch classifier, although it assumes homoscedasticity and so its performance depends on class covariance differences. This algorithm can be combined with Adaptive Margin Fisher's Criterion (AMFC) and Maximum Margin Criterion (MMC) to reduce the computational cost and solve the Small Sample Size (SSS) problem, hence, AMFC-LDA could accurately recognize faces on pose variations and unusual lighting conditions. Moreover, Independent Component Analysis (ICA) is a generalization of PCA, and has a set of vectors with maximum statistical independence; a recent variant is the natural logarithm based ICA algorithm (Log-LCA), which applies the natural logarithm in order to increase non-gaussianity and satisfies ICA's basic principle of separation; this combined with a classifier was robust when recognizing noisy face images [58].

Smart wearables provide physiological parameters such as: Electrocardiography (ECG), Electroencephalography (EEG), Heart Rate Variability (HRV), Electrodermal Activity (EDA), Respiration (RSP), Skin Temperature (SKT), Electromyography (EMG), among others, to predict emotion recognition, and required some of the methods previously mentioned: LDA, SVM, K-nearest neighbors (KNN) and Artifial Neural Network (ANN) [145]. This was comparable to the methods used by an example of a mHealth application, which implemented a multi-model prediction schema to predict four different classifiers of Asthma using Asthma Control Status (ACD) measurements, via models such as the well-known SVM, in addition to techniques that use classification trees (which are essentially a collection of binary trees): Random Forest and AdaBoost; the system provided the user chronic disease self-management capability [268].

Deep learning is becoming a popular method on classification problems, it re-assembles how the human brain works by creating a net of interconnected neurons, in which each neuron get a task, i.e., eye identification or mouth identification, in order to classify a bigger problem such as whole face recognition, in fact, there was a recent study in face recognition which used a Sparse Representation Classifier (SRC) to represent test data as a linear combination of training data by solving a L1-minimization, although the approach was sensitive to misalignment or a cropped face image, so a two-layered Convolutional Neural Network (CNN) feature extractor solved that problem because of its shift-invariant property [97]. Even so, fingerprint recognition could be also achieved via a deep neural network (DNN) using three hidden layers, stacked sparse auto-encoders and two classification probabilities for fuzzy classification, which provided higher accuracy than other methods which do not used Deep Learning structures [547]. Similar to the last approach, a CNN using low-powered wearable biosensors was capable of diagnosing arrhythmia using binary and quinary classifications, with remarkable accuracy $\geq 96.83\%$ [384].

When talking about behavioral recognition, it is important to state that each person has unique types of behavioral traits, for example: *(a)* Walking gait, *(b)* Touch gestures, *(c)* Keystroke dynamics, and many others [504]. This type of information can be used to identify a user with a similar approach to which physiological recognition works, wherein data is first extracted, then it passes to a pre-processing stage and finally for model fitting, though there are differences in the type of the data and the algorithms used.

User authentication is possible using behavioral patterns, mobile devices are usually integrated with sensors including an accelerometer, magnetometer and gyroscope, from which features such as: local X, Y, Z axes, the device acceleration, ambient geomagnetic field and rate of rotation are extracted [24]. These sensors are key on behavioral recognition and so by hand waving, they detect these features and a further method such as SVM or Random Forest Classifier is used in order to authenticate a person just by hand waving [504]. Authentication can be done via gait recognition, a novel Multi Kernelled Bijection Octal Pattern (MK-BOP) of extracted features from the signal generated by gait and applies a hybrid feature selector, including ReliefF (IRF) and Neighbor Component Analysis (NCA) to find the best discriminant, soon authenticating the user [38]. A similar approach was taken identifying eighteen classes of bird sounds, this was done via a multilevel Ternary Pattern (TP) and IRF classification method using SVM [527]. Additional research was done on gait analysis using Density-Based Spatial Clustering of Applications with Noise (DBSCAN), combined with a further K-means clustering method [547]. On the other hand, ECG, HRV and EGG signals with a Gaussian mixture model (GMM), and a SVM could asses psychological stress states using a new indicator Stress Classification Coefficient (SCC) [593]. Finally, deep learning networks (DNN) in combination of Hidden Markov Models (HMMs) and Gaussian Mixture Models (GMMs), classified 2-class and 4-class pathological speech and autism spectrum conditions, however, these deep architectures performed similar to the methods aforementioned such as Random Forest and SVM [115].

Moving on to voice recognition, Mel-Frequency Cepstral Coefficients (MFCC) are a widely used feature in this field; they are a variant of cepstral features using mel filter banks, which transforms the frequency bands so that they are equally spaced, with the objective of resembling a human auditory system's response. However, these coefficients are sensitive to noise, so pre-processing techniques have to be applied to the available data, then an additional method is usually implemented to select features related to speech recognition. Some studies that use MFCC to identify the speaker include: *(a)* Unique Mapped Real Transform (UMRT) to extract features and a Multi-layer perceptron ANN to classify [31], *(b)* Inner Hair Cell Coefficient (IHC) with Gaussian Mixture Model (GMM) and i-vector probabilistic models to acquire high accuracy among many other tested models [1]. A recent comprehensive study on Speech Emotion Recognition (SER) even combines IRF, MFCC, Human-Factor Cestral Coefficients (HFCC), including other techniques as a novel triangular filter bank, to create new filter banks (TFB-B and TFB-E), and so extract new variants of cepstral features (TFBCC-B and TFBCC-E), finally it used a SVM to classify the emotion of a speaker [356].

1.3.4 Commercial technology

The commercial technology for biometric systems can be divided into: non wearable and wearable systems. Non wearable technology includes those fixed systems, i.e., people assist the location of the equipment to be *sensed*. All those systems are laboratory equipment, medical, industrial and robotic platforms. These biometric systems have been the typical ones till the end of the last century.

With the arrival of the new century and the rise of electronic miniaturization Wearable technology has appeared. It uses biometric monitoring devices, which are sensors embedded in smartphones, wrist bands, skin patches, chest bands, headsets, or everyday objects that offer the opportunity to collect physiological, or behavioral personal data, continuously, remotely, and unobtrusively, [408].

1.3.4.1 Wearable biometrics

Data analysis and some affordable wearables, are a great way of directly helping people in preventing diseases or even treating them; a simple example is a method that requires an application on an Android Phone that manages a user's physiological parameters and a personal health file, that combined with PPG (Photoplethysmography) signals could create a dynamic monitoring of blood oxygen saturation as a method for the prevention and treatment of chronic cardiovascular disease [95]. There has also been a reduction in the number of wearables needed so that the user can feel natural wearing them; this is the case of gait predicting algorithms, which usually require many straps or adhesives attached to the person in question, although recent algorithms need only a wearable on a limb to predict macro gait with a high accuracy [188]. Recently, wrist-worn devices (WDDs) are becoming popular as they are affordable and helpful to the user, and so nowadays there are a variety of devices that can track a person's activity, as well as many other health related parameters, but

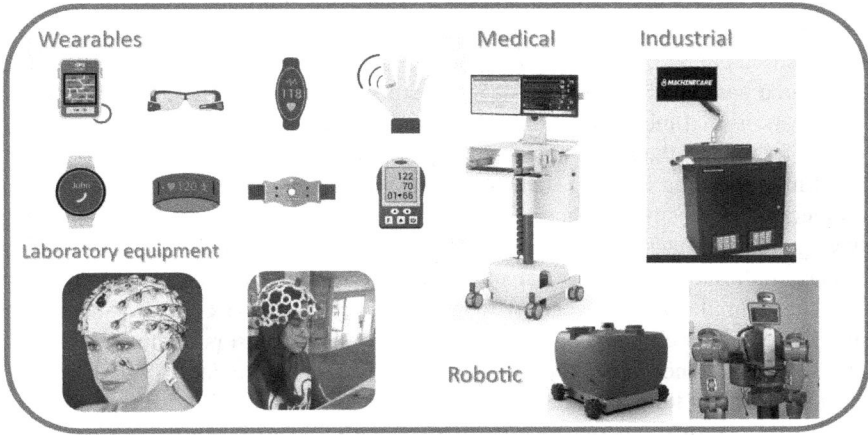

FIGURE 1.6: Commercial technology for biometric applications.

how reliable are they? A comparative study which included smartphones and smart watches from Samsung, Apple, Xiaomi, as well as fitness trackers such as diverse Fitbit and Garmin models, used a Bland-Altman method which showed that expensive and popular devices correlate with good accuracy predictions compared to the ground truth, which was acquired via an ECG when evaluating the effectiveness of hearth rate (HR), as well as an observer counting the number of steps using a tally counter [390].

Wearables can help people in self-management, with integrated machine learning algorithms, the devices providing measures with $\geq 90\%$ accuracy, which was the case with ECG and HR measures at slow walking speeds [295]; this parameter is crucial to monitor some chronic conditions such as Type 2 Diabetes (T2D) [241]. The predictions aforementioned also achieve results with similar accuracy on predicting sleep depth compared to clinical polysomnography (PSG) in adults [123], but also on adolescents with an additional actigraphy validation [291]. Although, based on the past studies, WDDs could not replace clinical devices as a diagnosis tool, because they became inaccurate in certain conditions, i.e., predicting HR when users are going fast at speeds more than 2.5 mph or 1.12 ms^{-1} [347], likewise predicting sleep, algorithms report both high and low sensitivity [198]. This suggests that WDDs are not to be taken as a ground truth, as many users suffer from consequences of doing so, as they may rely too much on a device and fortuitously self-diagnose a problem using *only* wearables [457]. With the rapid development of this technology, it is becoming infeasible for regulators to validate the functionality and security of each new wearable sensor, in spite of their high accuracy and results providing beneficial information to the user, medical devices are still considered as the ground truth of diagnosis. It is important to consider that, While designing WDDs, industries have to make a trade-off on a variety of factors including: commodity, accurate predictions, battery life and many other parameters, conversely medical devices diagnose accurately even when a patient has specific conditions. However, WDDs provide the user enough information to track self and perform better each day relative to a measurement, i.e., increasing the number of steps walked each day [328]. Another measured parameter by WDDs is energy expenditure, yet a recent review of multiple publications that included the brands mentioned at the beginning, concluded that no brand fell within the acceptable accuracy limits [173].

Smart clothing is being addressed with infants and elderly, which are common vulnerable groups in healthcare because of many reasons; there has been recent investigation that uses this technology to assist these groups. In the case of infants, recent studies using commercial smart socks for infants "Owlet Smart Sock", found out that cumulative incidence of tachyarrhythmia using HR monitors, was higher than detected by clinicians [28], while novel wireless sensors compatible with low-cost mobile phones showed performance equivalent to standard-of-care monitoring systems in premature neonates for high-income countries [570]. Likewise for the elderly, 3D designed customized smart shoes with Global Positioning System (GPS) and Radio Frequency Identification (RFID) provided not only satisfactory foot wear designs, but also safety services, to which parameters as HR, oxygenation level and many other parameters could be further implemented [263]. Industries are creating clothing to *(a)* improve exercises: Sensoria Fitness Socks for walking, Nadi X yoga pants to correct a pose, *(b)* Protect the user: Under Armour's Athlete Recovery reflecting heat as far as infrared light, Neviano Swimsuits to detect UV levels. On the other hand, research has been made with smart jackets measuring parameters such as pulse rate, sugar levels, blood pressure, biochemical oxygen demand (BOD) and others, using internal and external sensors, programmed via Lab VIEW [247].

Moreover, energy harvesting is popular nowadays, mainly because wearables require power, and so there has been a focus on developing clothing and wearables that can convert the heat generated by the human body to energy via thermoelectric generators (TEGs), however, the levels of power are still very low with regard to the energy that current devices and applications use [370]. Still, there has been recent improvement on creating flexible TEGs using Bi-Sb-Te screen-printing with no sign of degradation after a thousand bending cycles [81], as well as injekt printing of nanocomposite semiconductors $TiS_2(HA)_x$ [162]. Even if this technology is not sufficient for the current user needs and applications, with enough further research, it could be a technology that might solve many of commercial wearables' problems. On the other hand, smart glasses are being used for educational purposes in neurointerventional training, although there is not enough evidence that technology works for actual telemedicine [327]. However, there are recent studies showing its feasibility and acceptance when used by neurosurgery residents and specialists, which showed good to excellent internal consistency in addition to satisfaction with the method conducting ward rounds for neurocritical care patients during the recent COVID-19 pandemic [353].

1.3.4.2 Laboratory biometric systems

A traditional approach in physical biometrics is using physiological signals obtained from devices such as: electrocardiogram (ECG) from the heart, skin conductance (SC), electromyogram (EMG) from the muscles and electroencephalogram (EEG) from the brain; these are devices that measure the signals stated above using electrodes positioned on specific limbs across the body. There are numerous studies that use these devices, mainly because of their high accuracy and precision, thus the features can be used in order to detect different levels of stress among individuals [409], and so explore electrophysiological mechanisms of stress-induced arrhythmia [284]. The previous parameter was related with heart rate variability (HRV) during laboratory-based psychosocial stress, and on top of that, it has also shown sex differences [204]. On the other hand, stress can also be analyzed via derived heart rate signals from functional Near-Infrared Spectroscopy (fNIRS), or commonly refered as HRF [200], and it can provide measurements to classify autism spectrum disorders (ASDs) with respect to typically developed individuals (TDs) using fluctuation entropy, which quantifies the pattern diversity of a time series [568]. Moreover, a recent novel method used the VIVO 12-lead system software (Cathether Precision, Ledgewood, New Jersey), which is an electrocardiographic imaging (ECGi) device, combined with a cardiac magentic resonance (CMR) to create a tridimensional (3D) photograph of a patient's chest, to identify the most likely site of monomorphic ventricular tachycardia (VT) origin [362].

Posture and gait are features which are correlated to a person with diabetic polyneuropathy (DPN), as these parameters deteriorate depending on the severity of the illness. Features such as: foot height, step length, and stride length are associated with clinical and electrophysiological parameters retrieved from a nerve conduction study (NCS), thereafter the neurological status of these patients can be assessed via posture and gait [473]. Moreover, gait can be assesed using kinetic data from force plate strikes, followed by the Gait Deviation Index (GDI) calculation, which draw a correlation across pediatric patients with X-linked hypophosphatemia (XLH) [342].

With regard to sleep analysis, polysomnography (PSG) is usually considered as the gold standard, because it monitors many relevant body parameters accurately during sleep, such as: *(a)* Brain activity (EEG), *(b)* Eye movements (EOG), *(c)* Muscle activity (EMG), *(d)* Heart rhythm (ECG). There are a vast amount of studies that used PSG in order to find different sleep architectures among individuals, for example: *(a)* ASDs with respect to TDs [96], *(b)* depressed medicated adolescents within an inpatient pedopsychiatric unit [63], *(c)* suicidal ideation (SI) in treatment-resistant depression (TRD) [54]. As it was described before, PSG uses many devices, and so it tends to be costly, as well as time-consuming. Even though it is considered as the gold standard tool for sleep analysis in a sleep laboratory, other reliable methods are being explored, such as a combination of polygraphy (PG), pulse oximetry (SPO_2) and transcutaneous carbon dioxide pressure $P(tcCO_2)$, which was considered to be a valuable alternative for obstructive sleep apnea (OSA) evaluation in robin sequence (RS) infants, and thus diagnose obstructive sleep apnea syndrome (OSAS) [112].

Moving on to imaging, a recent method for Positron Emission Tomography (PET) used pure PET images to reduce partial volume effect (PVE), which is a common problem in PET imaging due to it's limited resolution. The method developed was done via an iterative deconvolution and shearlet transform, which in fact showed significant correction in terms of Myocardium Metabolic Rate for Glucose (MM-RGlu) [242]. Diffusion Tensor Imaging (DTI), is a complex non-invasive magnetic resonance imaging technique based on the diffusion of water in tissue, mostly used in neurology to provide a tridimensional (3D) image of the brain's neural track. An analysis of these images using a PCA revealed that brain diffusivity could in fact be used to identify a specific individual [512]. Likewise, three different modalities of magentic resonance imaging (MRI), combined with methods based on sparse matrix representations, were capable of creating a unique fingerprint among individuals. This was the result of high-resolution on cortical maps and connectors, which are unique for each individual [279].

Recent iris recognition studies explored whole eye axial biometry using Ultra-long Scan Depth Optical Coherence Tomography (UL-OCT). A study measured: anterior chamber depth (ACD), lens thickness, vitreous length, and axial length (AL) on a baseline during accommodation, which is a process made by the lens that lets the eye focus on nearby objects. After the accommodative stimuli (+6 D) was applied, the whole eye axial biometry changed, thus the device might be useful for full eye biometry during accomodation [591]. Alternatively, another study compared the accuracy of the recent intraoperature waverfront aberrometry (ORA) with respect to the Hill-radial basis functions (RBFs) in intraocular lens power selection, and found out that ORA best predicted residual refractive error and reduced hyperopic outcomes [219].

Genes are considered as a traditional biometric for human identification, mainly based on short tandem repeat (STR) markers of a DNA chain in order to profile an individual. Besides, recent studies have been designing a Human Identification Barcode System (HIBS) using DNA obtained by running PCR amplified products on agarose gel electrophoresis [581]. Moreover, denaturing high-performance liquid chromatography (DHPLC) has shown high levels of efficacy on forensic medicine characterizing D18S51 STR loci fragment, which is used for identity detection. The novel technique could perform DNA analysis for early screening of STRs at lower costs compared to capillary electrophoresis (CE) [154]. In addition, an alternative to the commonly used STR method was developed, which proposes the digitalization of a 72-plex single-nucleotide polymorphisms (SNPs). The technique in particular is designed so that it could be complex enough to identify everyone in the world, assigning a genetic identification number (GIN) to each digitalized SNP [179].

1.4   Trends

Some of the current trends are outlined in the following.

1.4.1 Connected systems

The integration of communication technologies into biometric systems allow to create networks of interconnected devices which can help to monitor and transfer biometric information for different purposes.

Some applications of connected biometric systems reported include multi-modal biometric systems [323], [450], cloud-centered biometric web services [252], low-cost security and authentication protocols [465], sensor operability [430], and human activity monitoring [183]. Healthcare applications of connected biometric systems also exist in the literature [239], [271].

In [239], an intelligent biometric system for elderly care was developed using a smart wristband, machine learning models, mobile computing and IoT protocols. The smart wristband was used to provide caretakers information on heart rate, temperature and motion of the patients, and a Hidden Markov Model (HMM) provided context awareness using such features as input. Combining this type of system with Big Data analytics would help to develop systems that allow to monitor multiple patients, record their information and build more reliable models [239].

Multimodal biometric systems are those that analyze a combination of multiple biometric features instead of only one [450]. Implementations of multimodal biometric systems represent more complex systems as they integrate different types of information and different methods are needed depending on the inputs. In order to develop these types of models, the information provided by different biometric recordings must be connected through a common node. Therefore, in a sense, these systems represent a network that integrates and interprets a combination of biometric descriptors [323]. Simple, yet effective low-cost multimodal biometric matching models can also be implemented such as the one presented in [465] using a Raspberry Pi and web Azure cloud.

A recent trend, integrating communication technologies and cloud services oriented to biometric systems has been defined as Internet of Biometric Things (IoBT) [252]. In [252], an application for the IoBT concept is proposed, which aims to add biometric information into the cloud for personal use such as more reliable authentication protocols which include GPS information, biometric recognition, thus providing context awareness as well. The use of IoT has also been described to find opportunities into smart cities, transportation and logistics, personal and social activities, agriculture and pharmaceutical industry [372].

1.4.2 Digital twins

Digital Twin technology has been addressed previously as one of the top trends in strategic technology in the recent years [458]. A Digital Twin is a virtual representation trying to emulate as closely as possible the parameters of a real, physical model of an object or process. The motivation of a Digital Twin is to provide reliable predictions based on previous knowledge of the parameters of the real model, and can also be used for intelligent decision making, monitoring and analysis [91].

While many applications of Digital Twins lie in the manufacturing industry, using biometric data such as medical records, fitness activity, lifestyle and nutritional information can provide insight to users, and they can be useful to predict possible risks, design personalized nutrition plans and training schedules, and make risk management evaluations at home and in the workplace [592].

Among many applications, some main areas of development in Biometrical Digital Twins have been identified in Behavioural, Human body, Sports and Healthcare Digital Twins.

1.4.2.1 Behavioral

Social media like Facebook and Instagram's algorithms are able to adapt to the content each user likes depending on their moods, temporal and fixed interests, friends and social activity such as texting, games and interactions with other users [148]. This feature applies to web services such as YouTube, Google and Amazon.

In a sense, all the information gathered in these platforms, fed by the same users, acts as a mirror of ourselves, and thus are able to propose content and profiles that might be of interest to the users [260]. Based on social media activity, researchers have been able to create personality prediction models using deep learning techniques fed with social activity records [508]. Thus, this is one step of a behavioral Digital Twin, that is able to provide to a certain extent, a virtual representation of the individual's personality. This type of model needs a bigger variety of data that describes behavioral traits, however, as algorithms and databases continue to grow, such models will become more and more reliable.

Another popular concept of a behavioural digital twin is that of Biometric daemons, virtual pets that accompany users, which are nurtured from them and learn personal traits from them to achieve a robust identity authentication [74]. In a sense, such pets learn their partner's fixed (fingerprint, iris) biometrics and then gain continuous experience through their "fluid" biometrics (voice, gait).

1.4.2.2 Human body

Digital Twins of the human body have different applications in the scientific literature. Digital twins of body organs, such as the heart [463] and its vessels [358] can help to save a considerable amount of resources by preventing unnecessary surgeries, excessive treatments, minimizing errors and avoiding risks in the medical field. One example of a Digital Twin of a heart is the *Living Heart Project* (https://www.3ds.com/products-services/simulia/solutions/life-sciences/the-living-heart-project/), a finite-element simulation of the heart, highly attractive for medical training in heart surgery.

Three-dimensional models of the human body can also be obtained by using scanning technologies to map the reality into a virtual representation. One example is described in [463], where such a model was achieved through advanced image processing of multiple Kinect devices capturing a human body from different angles. These type of models can be used for entertainment applications, such as creating virtual avatars modelled after their users' bodies; while they can also be useful for fitness and medical purposes.

1.4.2.3 Sports

The use of virtual technology has been expanding across different fields with a positive impact. Sports science is one such, as digital solutions provide more precise, accurate and timely information about athletic performance [447]. A Digital Twin using biometric records has also been reported in the literature for fitness purposes [48]. In this work, biometric data from athletes was gathered in 22 features, including sleep quality, gait behaviour, food income, caloric intake and mood. Statistical and machine learning methods were used to identify the most relevant features and a predictive model was designed to predict performance during training, and if necessary, made suggestions on the athletes' behaviour.

1.4.2.4 Healthcare

Customization has been one of the most important features in health care service from the past decades. The use of IoT, communication technology and web services have facilitated this process due to fast information interchange. The development of Digital Twins in healthcare shows promise across different levels: patient, health system, health and treatment goals, biometric monitoring, technology and wellness [458].

Healthcare and well-being services can not only be of interest to hospitals. Such Digital Twins can also benefit industries, as it would help to track the employers' health state, which could be useful for early prevention and treatment, as well as risk reduction. Digital Twins in healthcare can also be used to construct data-driven personalized medical services for each user, and have also been proposed as human enhancement technologies, due to their predictive and intelligent decisive component [75].

One main consideration is the need of data to construct the virtual models. Two approaches can be considered: Big and Small Data. While Big Data focuses on gathering information from many databases and records that help to create more reliable and general models; Small Data focuses on personalized models, fed with information from the same patient [458]. As a summary, the use of biometrics in the development of virtual representations of the human have a lot of potential across different fields, and will continue to arise in the next years.

1.4.3 Smart communities

As technology continues to expand across the world, the concept of "smartness" has reached different components of our lives, such as smart phones, smart watches, smart cars and more recently, smart cities and communities [29]. Smart communities refer to the intelligent use of technologies for the benefit of different aspects of communities such as optimized resource and waste management [391], increased connectivity [276], accessibility to services [52], data transparency [71], smart government [197], and security [150], among other many examples.

Smart communities' deployments are characterized by the use of connected services, data transfer, sensors and communication technologies [209]. Within the smart community framework, there also exists the concept of the smart citizen, which is the user of all the available technologies and makes use of them to its fullest capability to enhance their everyday life experiences. In order to provide the best experience to its citizens, cities and communities must be able to provide customizable services such as entertainment and retail.

In our current age, services offered to consumers are customizable to a certain extent with the use of predictive models based on social media, streaming platforms, and web services' activity [186]. Such customization could be further enhanced by including the use of behavioural and physiological biometrics into this framework. Biometric applications are more and more often implemented in everyday life activities such as fitness and health, and this trend is assured to continue. A very recent trend called Biometrics as a Service (BaaS) has been promoting the use of biometric applications and their accessibility to all kinds of users and fields [45].

Biometrics in the smart community represent an inclusion of physiological and behavioural data of citizens, which could be used for better decision taking and options in:

1. Personalized healthcare services: The use of medical records and their ease of access to physicians and medical personnel can allow to speed up and optimize diagnoses, treatment and follow-up [576]. This same context applies in insurance services, work-related medical tests and examinations.

2. Personalized services and entertainment activities: The use of emotion detection, obtained through video and/or wearable sensors' data analysis, can increase the information about human experiences and reactions to different services or entertainment options. This could lead to optimized suggestions on preferred activities and services, which is highly valuable for marketing purposes [307].

3. Personalized retail services: Access to data such as gender, age, weight, height, and anatomical data can be useful for citizens/stores to make better choices when buying/selling garments, footwear, sportswear, accessories, products for sense augmentation/restoration (e.g., glasses, hearing aid devices), among many other options [163].

4. Education services: The use of behavioural and physiological biometrics can greatly enhance learning by providing feedback to students or educators about students' personalities, emotions, reactions, cognitive and physical state, personal and collaborative preferences, teamwork synergy and mood [122].

5. Connectivity and social media: Social Behavioral Biometrics (SBB) can be extracted from social media activities such as social interactions, game

preferences, and content sharing. Additionally, inclusion of physiological biometrics such as *natural* emotions, fitness information, and audiovisual recordings could enhance this experience and connectivity to other users [506].

It is important to consider that in all the aforementioned applications, data sharing and access is a must. In this regard, some users are reluctant to this type of technology, mostly due to data privacy distrust [176]. This is understandable, as not all users would be comfortable or willing to share content about their physiological or behavioural data.

Such distrust could be alleviated as time passes and the use of biometrics spreads across the world and becomes more popular among citizens. A similar case is that of identity recognition through biometrics for humanitarian purposes, which started around early 2000's in border agencies and twenty years later is a well-known and wide spread technology [231]. However, time by itself is not sufficient to solve this distrust among users. Therefore, data privacy and security is a very important aspect that needs to be considered when performing BaaS deployments in Smart Communities.

1.5 Applications

1.5.1 Health

Biometric technology for healthcare applications has gained much interest over the last years due to its diverse applications, not only for security or accessibility purposes but also for diagnosis and effective treatment [324]. Patient records are very delicate information; their loss could mean the administration of an erroneous treatment, and they can also be used for malicious purposes if accessed by the wrong people [343]. The use of biometric traits as a means of identification to protect patient databases has become a popular alternative [595, 213], particularly since electronic records are being adopted by many institutions [213]. Not only does it improve the security of the system and requires less effort from the user, but it can also reduce prices related to password maintenance [595].

Insurance companies are also taking advantage of biometrics to avoid scams [324, 382]. This offence costs up to 30 billion dollars annually in the US [427]. By applying a recognition system, these companies could avoid charges for illegitimate health services, including treatments not given, already paid for or not necessary [382]. Also, in case of an emergency, patients can be identified even if they were not carrying an ID card [595], increasing their chances to survive.

Wearable sensors are extensively used for non-invasive diagnosis and monitoring of several medical conditions. Heart activity and blood pressure can be acquired using PPG or ECG sensors, although the second type is more reliable for accurate diagnosis [537] and the first type is used for recording during daily activities [86].

Nevertheless, the simplicity of operation, wearing comfort for patients and cost effectiveness of PPG technology has motivated researchers to develop more accurate devices, and modern devices have the potential to replace ECG recordings [64]. Some cardiovascular diseases that can be diagnosed with the use of biometric sensors include atherosclerosis, hypertension, and arrhythmias [86]. If combined with other sensors, such as temperature, humidity or pulse oximetry, the blood pressure can also be used to monitor patients suffering from chronic respiratory or kidney diseases and determine the need for medications or specialized medical attention [130, 556].

Other biological signals have also been proposed for healthcare applications. Electrodermal activity (EDA) can be used to detect epileptic seizures before they happen [404], or to detect distress conditions to ensure mental health [582]. The combination of EDA and heart rate variability can predict the emotional response of autistic children, improving their development and serving as a communication tool with their parents [275]. Gait analysis can be used to detect posture instability [155], but the most common use is to monitor the elderly and alert in case of a fall [499] or during daily activities, allowing them to live independently [77].

The inclusion of various sensors into commercial devices, such as smartwatches, has also improved the promotion of a healthier lifestyle by encouraging people to exercise more and take care of their body [259]. The accessibility to this kind of technology can also help smokers keep track of their cigarette consumption with the use of the watch's accelerometers, and instead engage them with behaviour changing techniques [489].

1.5.2   Education

Schools stand to benefit from biometric technology in several ways. Logistically speaking, the implementation of biometric scanners that enable students to have immediate access to facilities such as library withdrawals, gymnasiums, transportation services, or cafeteria accounts through which to handle their meal payments have already been implemented, and are commercially available through companies such as IDconnect, identiMetrics and M2SYS [181]. Despite this, the level of acceptance is not clear, given that some countries embrace the technology and some have put up legal walls to prevent the implementation of biometrics in academic contexts [290], [318].

For the aforementioned applications, the parameters used are mostly facial recognition through cameras and fingerprint identification [181], [290]. In the context of education per se, the main goal of biometrics is to identify and measure the cognitive state of alumni, be it through identification of engagement, boredom, cognitive load, attention, and concentration [258]. Four distinct categories of biometrics are used in combination to achieve this.

1.5.2.1   Neural imaging

Consequently, neuroimaging techniques such as fMRI and EEG have been considered; fMRI offers high quality data that can be used to visualize even on a problem from a set of exercises a student is working on [25], but comes with a price tag that makes it inaccessible to most. EEG, on the other hand, offers lower quality information, but at a lesser price and an increased ease-of-use. Since EEG signals can be analyzed in different frequency bands which are in turn related to mental and emotional states, it has been used to identify if the user is paying attention to the intended target [72]. In fact, it has been shown that giving direct feedback on their concentration level to students can help improve their learning pace and retention [193].

1.5.2.2 GSR

The galvanic skin response (GSR) has also been explored as a means to achieve this. Through GSR, methodologies to assess individual willingness and degree of comfort when working with mates on projects and presentations have been proposed and demonstrated as feasible [121], [120]. Other signals identified as indicators of focus and attention are HRV, blood pressure (BP) and interheart intervals [519], [516], [540]. Despite there being evidence that each of these signals might be reliable on its own, such as the relationship between HRV and college freshman final exams performance [519], the tendency is to integrate as many inputs as possible to the biometric classifiers. The reasoning behind this is that no single parameter is directly and exclusively related to any of the intended identification states. The current body of literature suggests that the use of several sensors can yield exponentially better results in terms of reliability and accuracy, as exemplified by the combination of cardiac sensors, GSR sensors, and EEG equipment [516], [120].

1.5.2.3 Camera

Cameras are yet another sensor that yield a vast amount of information. Audio signals can be analyzed to detect who participates, and how their interactions relate to the class dynamics [121]. However, the main contribution of cameras lies in eye tracking and facial analysis. Eye tracking performed at a sampling frequency as low as 30 Hz has been shown to be useful, but 60 Hz has shown better results in classifying where on a screen the student is concentrating on [133]. Eye tracking measures two main parameters, eye fixation (for a specified time window) and saccades [565]; after due calibration, heat maps can be generated to indicate which regions of the screen attract the students gaze the most, if at all [503], [133]. Facial analysis can also help measure behavioural engagement [132]. It is also useful to catalog the emotional state of the student, which is useful to determine if the class he or she is in engaging him or not. Interestingly, the attention allocated by the students to specific content depends on factors such as prior knowledge of the topic, which hint at the potential for personalized adaptive learning strategies derived from these technologies [514].

1.5.2.4 Others

Lastly, some non conventional sensors have been proposed to identify the state of focus of the class such as pressure sensors to measure student comfort when seated [157]; the intention behind this is to determine if the furniture is comfortable enough as to allow the student to focus solely on the lecture. Further, thermal imaging for real time feedback to the instructor has been reported, as to best modulate the way he conducts the class based on the level of attention of the class and their collective emotional state [258].

1.5.3 Business

Business is yet another area into which biometrics have permeated due to the safe alternative they pose against conventional password identification and digital protection methods [16]. Just like other areas of application, biometric applications in business can be grouped into distinct fields of study. In this case, three main areas can be distinguished from current reported uses: biometrics as a service, financial services security, and workplace biometrics.

1.5.3.1 Biometrics as a service

Biometrics are, in essence, a series of mathematical operations performed on a set of biometric data to assess the probability of a condition being true, usually pertaining to identification of subjects. However, as the complexity of the software that carries out these operations increases, so does the computational cost. This has led to the offer of outsourcing these operations to online service providers [437] [46]. The advantage that biometrics has as a service (BaaS) is that cloud computing is already employed in both scientific and business activities [47]. In fact, one of the BaaS applications discussed in the literature consists of integrating a BaaS as an authentication alternative to passwords to access cloud-based data [47]. However, even the distribution of software itself to evaluate biometrics constitutes a BaaS. A main constraint on this business model is the computational load, but some proposals have already been identified as efficient low-cost (computational) protocols for biometric authentication [128].

1.5.3.2 Financial services user authentication

Although authentication of an individual through biometrics is a recurrent theme throughout this work, financial institutions have not yet fully adopted this technology despite its potential usefulness, such as increased adoption of biometrics amongst people between the ages of 24 and 16 years [369], or the fact that biometric factors such as vein biometrics are already employed for some financial transactions security factors [346].

Given the increased security need of financial institutions, a special focus on hard to replicate biometrics has been placed in current investigations [375], [76], [490]. One approach has been made towards securing access to bank information by generating a convolutional neural network that obtained a 93% accuracy rate on identification of facial features of individuals and comparing them to official pictures that had been previously submitted to the bank. A caveat for this approach is that the pictures in the bank's servers need to meet certain specific criteria for the model to be accurate enough [375].

Another idea that has been put forward is the identification of a user on a mobile device by considering two behavioral biometrics in combination by using the cadence of typing of a person along with the phone movements produced during the typing of the password. The strength of this proposed authentication mechanism is based not on the uniqueness of the biometrics, but rather on the difficulty of replication of the same [76]. Yet another feature that has been suggested is voice recognition as an additional means for user identification [490].

Despite the several areas of opportunity that biometrics have in the banking industry, the main barrier that they have yet to overcome prior to widespread adoption is ensuring security of users' data security. For example, some authors have reported amongst the strategies in place to protect sensible information simply by installing reliable antivirus software [37]. One issue that is yet to be addressed is the protection of the biometric templates, both if they are stored in the device or in a remote media [374], [306].

1.5.3.3   Workplace biometrics

The application of biometrics to the workplace has the potential to automate many monitoring and security authentication processes. For example, a system has been proposed such that it employs analysis of gait and posture, both behavioural biometrics, to track an employee within the boundaries of the employer's facilities to be able to offer insights in regard to the use of and personal flow inside the workplace [515]. Further, the use of biometrics can enhance the anthropometric knowledge of the user of a device, such as building and construction machinery, in terms of their posture and how the prolonged use of equipment affects their health, as so to improve the design of their tools [470].

Strongly related to the previous point, the attention of an operator of any device is of interest due to its impact on the productivity of the employee; because of this, nonobtrusive behavioural biometric tracking systems have been brought forward with the goal of identifying the level of concentration of the individual, such as mouse clicking and moving, typing cadence on a keyboard, and switching between two tasks [141].

Authentication of identity, a recurrent theme in this chapter, has useful carryover to the workplace too. Systems that serve as a two factor authentication to ensure that only qualified or intended users of a device have access to it such as tracking of eye movement and response to a series of images have been demonstrated as feasible [407]. On the same line of thought, a system based on identification of hand and arm gestures to generate secure personal pins have been proposed, [371] with the added benefit of needing no contact between the device and the user to validate identification, a feature that has gained relevance as a result of the recent COVID-19 pandemic.

Driving one step further towards automation of tracking processes and detection of possibly harmful activities and postures, such as a curved back while moving and lifting, or bad postures while sitting, a system was devised to be able to do this through a single sign-in. The value in this is that as employees enter and exit rooms, current systems require (often) a sign in is required when someone reenters the room again, which becomes tedious and is a friction point in the usability of the systems. By using IoT technology, a wearable sensor links to the user's phone and uses wifi to track the user in real time without the need for multiple sign-ins onto the system [589].

1.5.4   Marketing

Marketing can be considered separated from business applications given the different purposes of each. Marketing approaches, as is discussed in this section, focus on the categorization of the biometrics gathered from a customer or client in response to a stimulus, usually an ad or a product. There are two main areas of research regarding this topic, which are neuromarketing on the one hand, and non-neural biometrics on the other.

1.5.4.1   Neuromarketing

Although neuromarketing is sometimes used to refer to all biometric marketing, it is helpful as a first approach to differentiate between neural-oriented strategies and physiology-oriented data recollection. Biometric applications in marketing can be approached under the term of Neuro-marketing (NM), which focuses on measuring the effect of products and advertisements on a target audience. It should come as no surprise that NM efforts to quantify physiological responses to marketing stimulus employ EEG set-ups to record and process brain activity [224], [35], [573], [69], [18], [189], [199].

Various ways of accomplishing this have been proposed. For example, one route explored is to perform specific signal decomposition and analysis in either a time or frequency domain to observe specific phenomena associated with particular emotional states [189]. Alternatively, bandpass filters can be applied to obtain certain bandwidths, namely alpha, beta, theta and gamma, and ratios such as the frontal alpha asymmetry, related to preference states are calculated [18], [199]. Once this has been accomplished, data generated can be fed into artificial intelligence (AI) models to predict or classify the response of the user or target audience. Such models have proven to be successful in classifying the response in real time when the users are exposed to stimuli such as videos, travel agency web-pages and product packaging [18].

The use of EEG, and some other neuroimaging techniques [69] has been explored, but just as is the case of education applications, the constraints that such equipment place on the recollection of data have led investigators to consider alternative biometrics.

1.5.4.2   General biometrics

Emotions triggered by a product or service are strongly correlated with the customers' willingness to purchase or engage in multiple interactions with the vendor [289], [35], [224]. In order to exploit this, emotion processing, eye tracking and facial analysis have been proposed as viable alternatives to EEG. Furthermore, given the current ubiquity of cameras, which are embedded in almost every phone and computer made, offering a high degree of portability, enables marketers to forego previous limitations being able to analyze target audiences only in fixed locations, since they have a resolution high enough to allow for eye tracking [138]. Modern AI software that carries out facial coding and sentiment analysis has been key to the implementation of this biometric, since it enables marketers to obtain information from multiple potential customers without having to manually analyze each video or or facial picture taken [224], [246].

Eye tracking technology has been widely adopted as a biometric to map consumer preferences and attention allocation [69], [448]. There are models available commercially that track and analyze the movement of the eyes with respect to items on a screen through proprietary or open source software. To do this, the sensor is calibrated with a sequence of eye movements [138]. A study investigated the effect on the visual attention the user dedicated to different elements of an ad for infant products depending on whether the model faced the viewer sideways or directly. As it turned out, the audience focused more on the face of the model as opposed to the product when facing it [35].

Given the established relationship between eye movement and focus of attention, this measure has been used with GSR to determine which parts of a graphic resource elicited more intense emotions, since it can be used to determine relative levels of excitation due to sweat gland activity [333], [309], [203]. As well, GSR and pupillometry, the study of pupil size change in response to a stimulus, have been used in combination to analyze the effort of focusing on a region of interest on a screen [531], [424], [224].

Some other applications related to biometric marketing are thermal and 3D cameras that help identify the state of agitation of customers, and their reactions to products or services [226]. Posture as well has been correlated to the interest and intent for the purchases of test subjects [424], but more research is needed to determine if there is a direct correlation between the two. One more biometric application that is proposed in the current literature is nanobiometrics, which relies on the use of nanotechnology to gather multiple simultaneous streams of information while the subject of study carries out his daily life, thanks to the non-invasiveness of these sensors [339].

As mentioned in previous sections of this chapter, behavioural biometrics are an emerging field. In RFID marketing applications tagging has been used in real life stores to analyze the pattern of flow of products within the store, and segments the type of customers that arrive based on how they move with relation to them [285]. Further, text mining of social media as part of a sentiment analysis can yield valuable results with a minimum investment required on behalf of a business owner [360].

Both behavioural and traditional biometrics often make use of machine learning to make the analysis of the amount of information obtained from the information sources feasible. It is because of this that it is important to point out that feature selection for the computer models is a determinant factor in the effectiveness of the biometric tool, and that an optimal combination of input parameters must be achieved to yield satisfactory results [535], [246].

1.5.5   Industry

This section explores the use of Biometrics in industries. It mainly explores the reasoning behind its implementation in evolving businesses, and the benefits which are acquired through its implementation in business work models, and future research opportunities concerning this area. The biometry field has considerable applications in distinct industries (public and private) which have impacted day-to-day operations in an unprecedented way. The following topic will be divided into three sections:

1. How and why biometry has been applied in industries.

2. Biometric applications which have been proven to have an impact in industries and its workers.

3. Future research proposals and opportunities biometrics could have in industries.

1.5.5.1   How and why biometry has been applied in industries

As already detailed in this chapter, biometric technology can make use of either anatomical or physiological characteristics in a very precise manner (be it through fingerprints, heart rate, face images iris or retina visualization, hand geometry) or behavioral ones (written signatures, voice, keyboard typing patterns) [78]. to create individual signals that are personal to each user and can be measured and authenticated through biometric technology.

Industry leaders have shown an interest in the potential benefit of implementing biometric technology in their operations. Anatomical readings have proven to be of great value from both a security and data analysis standpoints [392]. A great recurrent example of the said phenomenon for authentication purposes would be enterprises using this technology to analyze certain employees' unique iris patterns [434]. The said patterns would be visualized and translated into a signal with an infrared camera mounted on an operating system that is able to link the said employee's unique and uncopiable data with a security clearance code to unlock a door and grant access to certain facilities [109].

However, the areas which have lately shown the most promise and growth in the industry are both behavioral and physiological biometry [89]. The said areas have the capacity to recollect information from users who use specialized wearable devices that monitor specific physiological signals (for example EEG or ECG signals) emitted during daily activities be it working out, clinical check-ups, in their workplace, or even while sleeping. It must be noted that these devices are considerably powerful given that they are capable of monitoring human performance continuously in environments that are outside a laboratory or clinic with ease. The said devices extract data from their users and consecutively input it into algorithms to analyze it and improve its user's quality of life [538]. Enterprises have realized that they can use this advantageously to improve their workers safety, health, and all-around quality of life [243]. This will be elaborated further in the following section.

1.5.5.2 Biometric applications which have been proven to have an impact on industries and their workers

Besides security, biometric technology has proven to be highly useful in industries for two specific purposes: ergonomics and employee wellbeing.

Ergonomics: Ergonomics is defined as the set of "Principles for optimization of human and overall system efficiency" [532]. This simply means that it is the scientific branch which looks to optimize worker productivity, efficiency, and safety while on the job. To measure and apply ergonomics, workplaces utilize sensor systems. The said systems consist of multiple sensors which are utilized in unison to obtain and analyze precise user information. Formerly, sensor systems were defined as: "a platform composed of different types and number of sensors, which are positioned in different locations on the body and whose signals are processed in parallel and combined to provide specific parameters in real-time" [500]. These systems help to analyze risk factors and thus improve work conditions. For example, Antwi-Afari developed a non-invasive method to automatically detect, classify and notify concerned parties about awkward working postures in construction workers based on foot planting pressure distribution data measured by a wearable insole pressure system which was inputted into a machine learning algorithm in MATLAB® [32].

Employee wellbeing: Biometric technology has demonstrated considerable uses in employee wellness programs to be able to upkeep and improve workers' mental and health conditions [389]. Successful programs typically consist of promoting healthy lifestyle choices and activities; however, it's been demonstrated that the most successful ones include a core component referred to as: Health risk identification tools. This component consists of technology tools (be it wearables, or any specialized IoT sensor) specialized in health risk assessments using biometric screenings which monitor relevant health variables such as body mass index, blood pressure, cholesterol and glucose levels and more. Industries have established that successful implementation of the previously mentioned applications (ergonomics and wellbeing) can improve working conditions, employee morale, and productivity. However, enterprises must always consider that optimal use adherence and outcomes largely depend on the task force's acceptance of the technology [230]. Research has shown that some employees resist utilizing this technology voicing concerns regarding privacy or confidentiality of the collected data, and compliance [453]. It is up to each of these industries and the scientific community to be able to adapt to these barriers and assure user privacy.

1.5.5.3   Future research proposals and opportunities

The biometric field has ample growth opportunities within industries. These vary from:

1. Robust matching: Improving the matching algorithm's performance in the presence of imperfect conditions (segmentation, noise, and inherent signal variance) [439].

2. Reference update: Updating references effectively and effortlessly so that they can account for variations and aging of reference data in long-lived systems (such as facial aging) [439].

3. Robustness in facing adversaries: Improving defenses against cyber-attacks, including protection from falsified biometric traits [439].

1.5.6   Sports

The biometric branch has demonstrated potential to keep athletes safer and healthier, while maximizing their training regimen and providing unprecedented insights about their performances [49]. Mark Gorski, co-founder and chief executive of Sports Data Labs, (a biometrics technology provider located in the US) has said that biometry "can help you train more efficiently or change the way you do things in a match" [49]. The following section will explore and elaborate upon the previous statement. It will be divided into three sections:

1. Biometric relevance in sports.

2. Biometric applications in sports and results.

3. Future research areas and important considerations.

1.5.6.1   Biometrics relevance in sports

Research has demonstrated there is a direct correlation between biometric technology utilization and injury prevention [299]. The said claims are a direct consequence of the growth in biometric technology which due to widespread adoption of wearable sensors and camera-kinetic analysis has facilitated human motion analysis [511]. Additionally, sports' scientists have made practical use of the quantitative data generated through these technologies and have been making performance assessment reports to heighten athlete performances [564].

1.5.6.2   Biometric applications in sports and results

Using wearable sensors and kinetic analysis are the most frequently practiced methodologies for monitoring and evaluating athletic activities. This section will be elaborating on how these methods work.

Wearable sensors: The ever-developing technology field has permitted wearable devices and sensors to be accessible to all classes of athletes be it individual endurance athletes, sport teams, or physicians, who are all interested in monitoring relevant biometric parameters which are fundamental to enhancing performance and minimizing injury. Movement sensors include pedometers, accelerometers or gyroscopes, and global positioning satellite (GPS) devices. Physiological sensors include heart rate and sleep monitors, temperature and integrated sensors [564], [460], [191].

All the obtained data and variables which are obtained through these sensors tend to be inputted into machine and deep learning models which have the capability to analyze athlete movements and habits and recognizing any potentially harmful irregularity requiring correction [116].

An example of this would be S. Saponara's work in designing an athlete performance measurement system for combat sports. The said system is utilized to measure training effectiveness and moves utilizing accessible, low-cost devices which have the capacity to operate in real time with algorithms and thus evaluate athlete performance be it their kick effectiveness, speed, power, stance, or other relevant variables [449].

Kinetic analysis: Kinetic analysis which focusses primarily on biomechanical variables is another tool for analyzing and assessing athlete performance in sports [124]. Video analysis and its effectiveness depend a lot on the complexity of the model. It can be done either manually by utilizing kinetic software platforms to select the position of the relevant body parts per frame in a video, or automatically through data visualization software and image recognition algorithms which automate this procedure [88]. The said algorithms consist of dynamic and complex analyses (i.e., non-linear Multi-Dimensional Scaling, classification and regression tree, logistic regression, and more) utilized for a deeper understanding of athlete performance [471].

This kinetic technology tends to be complemented with wearables and sensors. In unison, interested athletes, coaches, and evaluators, have become capable of developing deep and profound evaluations of athlete performance and areas of opportunity be it by maximizing biomechanical variables through proper stances /posture, or through observation systems[471]. For example, [525] developed an observational instrument which analyses tennis players' strokes. The said system calculates a total of 23 variables when a player strokes the ball. Through algorithms they are analyzed and displayed to any interested parties and lets them "evaluate their own actions and their opponents from a technical-tactical perspective", benefiting them to better their performance through an improvement in their training programs and analysis of the technical-tactical qualities of any impending rivals [525].

1.5.6.3 Future research areas and important considerations

There is ample room for biometric research and improvement within the sports industry. A major opportunity would be improving algorithmic accuracy and reliability. An example would be John Gleaves research. He has developed a biometric mathematical algorithm which analyzes a variety of hematological and steroidal markers from tests done on athletes and determines if any irregular fluctuations (at least naturally) indicate the use of performance enhancing drugs (PED's) [187]. However, much debate of the algorithm's accuracy and reliability still gets triggered which has led some organizations to discard utilizing the said doping analysis.

Another important factor which requires improvement is data protection and ethical considerations. Jason F. Arnold advocates that "federal regulations do not address the use of biometric technologies in sports" [34]. This basically means that sport organizations, (particularly from universities or high schools) should establish proper protocols and governing bodies in order to protect all the user data and privacy. Arnold finishes stating that "further research on the validity and interpretation of biometric data in amateur and professional sports is urgently needed and should include a more systematic approach for gathering information on the prevalence of biometric technologies and existing privacy protections[34], which clearly demonstrates that there is plenty of scope for growth within this field before it truly prospers [253].

1.6   Glossary

360 Degree Review: Performance review that includes feedback from superiors, peers, subordinates, and clients.

Abnormal Variation: Changes in process performance that cannot be accounted for by typical day-to-day variation. Also referred to as non-random variation.

Acceptable Quality Level (AQL): The minimum number of parts that must comply with quality standards, usually stated as a percentage.

Activity: The tasks performed to change inputs into outputs.

Adaptable: An adaptable process is designed to maintain effectiveness and efficiency as requirements change. The process is deemed adaptable when there is agreement among suppliers, owners, and customers that the process will meet requirements throughout the strategic period.

2

Analysis of Electrophysiological Activity of the Nervous System: Towards Neural Engineering Applications

Luz María Alonso-Valerdi

2.1 Bioelectrical human information

A biosignal is a signal coming from any living entity. This signal should be measurable, trackable and analyzable. A biosignal can be either electrical or non electrical. Biosignals have attributes (or features) that provide valuable information to investigate the physical (or even mental) condition of the living entity. In Figure 2.1, biosignals typically monitored on the human being are illustrated, both electrical and non electrical ones. The most monitored systems are: (1) cardiovascular (2) respiratory (3) peripheral and central nervous system (4) muscular and (5) dermal. Conventional recording techniques of biosignals are also summarized in Figure 2.1.

According to [264] biosignals do not vary randomly or arbitrary. Namely, brain and body signal oscillations are aligned with each other and form a single frequency architecture. The interaction between the brain and the body may be described as a complex system that couples and decouples according to a specific harmony frequency described by

$$f_d(i) = s * 2^i \tag{2.1}$$

where s is the scaling factor, i refers to the biosignal of interest, and f is the fundamental frequency of the biosignal oscillation. When i = 0, f_d refers to cardiac activity. When i $<$0, f_d refers to breathing rhythms (including Mayer waves having the lowest frequencies in the respiratory process), blood pressure (BP) waves, rhythmic fluctuations in the blood oxygen level dependent (BOLD) signal at intrinsic mode fluctuations (IMD), and gastric waves. When i $>$0, f_d refers to brain oscillations.

Besides, upper and lower frequencies of each fundamental frequency can be respectively estimated by

$$uf_d(i) = \frac{1.25 \times 2^{i+1}}{g} \tag{2.2}$$

$$lf_d(i) = (1.25 \times 2^{i-1}) \times g \tag{2.3}$$

Tecnologico de Monterrey.

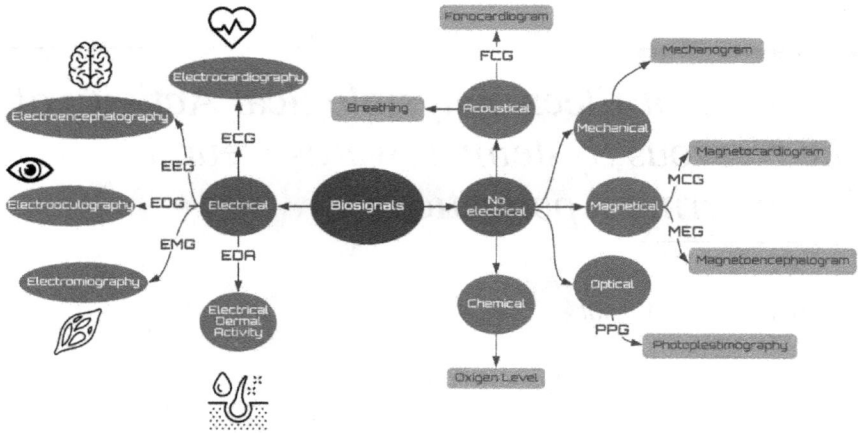

FIGURE 2.1: Biosignals of the human being. Human functioning depends on cell communication that is based on (but not limited to) the transmission of electrical currents through the tissues. Such current transmission generates magneto-electrical fields, and can be reflected as sound, motion, oxygen level modification, and even, impedance and temperature changes. This is why several types of biosignals, either electrical or non electrical, can be measured on the human body.

In Figure 2.2, frequency bands of the biosignals are calculated according to the brain-body coupling theorem for an individual with 75 beats per minute (s = 1.25 Hz). This theorem demonstrates that resonance of a biosignal is harmonized with other signals, and then, the same information may be obtained from different sources to design biometry technology. For instance [265],

- During respiration, heart rate increases during inhalation and decreases during exhalation.

- Heart rate presents a clear tendency 10:1 frequency ratio relative to breathing rate owing to energy demands and emotional regulation.

- Gastric waves explain 8% of the alpha band modulations of EEG signals, and 15% of the BOLD variance is explained by the gastric phase.

- Slow frequency that modulates the envelope of the EMG signal originates from neural mechanisms of motor control and resonance frequencies of body parts.

2.1.1 Electrophysiological activity of the nervous system

Human beings have three main electrical sources: (1) neurons, (2) cardiac cells and (3) muscles. Electrical activity reflects the functionality of the Nervous System, both Central (CNS) and Peripheral (PNS). The typical recording technique of the CNS is Electroencephalography (EEG). On the other hand, the PNS can be monitored

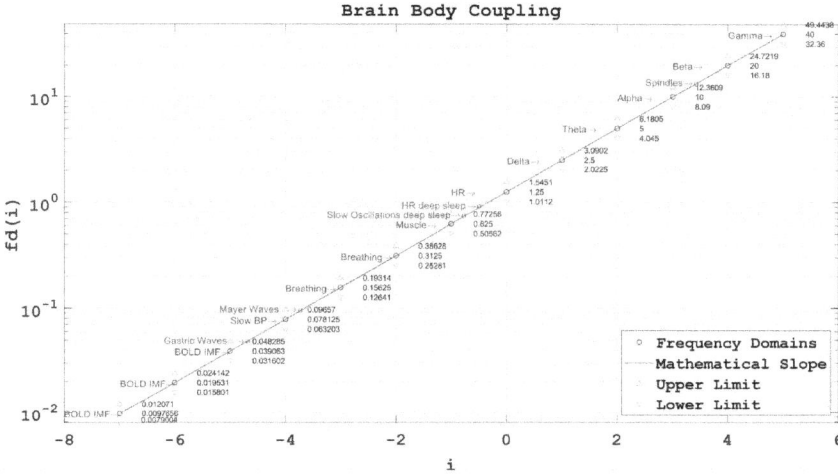

Brain Body Coupling

FIGURE 2.2: Brain-body coupling theorem postulated in [2] and applied to an individual with 75 beats per minute. Positive integers determine brain oscillations, whereas negatives ones define breathing, BP, BOLD and gastric waves. Zero refers to cardiac activity at rest.

through Electromyography (EMG) and Electrooculography (EOG) for the somatic system, and Electrocardiography (ECG) and Electro-dermal Activity (EDA) for the autonomous one. Somatic and autonomous PNS are involved in the voluntary and involuntary control of the human body respectively. The main electrical features of all these electrophysiological signals are outlined in Table 2.1. So far, the analysis of the electrical activity of the human body has aimed at six main purposes:

- Cognitive applications: To analyze the processing of information in the human being.

- Social applications: To study relationships in terms of cognition, emotions and behavioral patterns.

- Developmental applications: To investigate psychological development and the aging process.

- Environmental applications: To find interconnections among individuals, technologies and contexts.

- Clinical applications: To give an insight into neuronal disorders.

- Practical applications: To propose and improve bio- and neuro-feedback approaches.

TABLE 2.1: Electrophysiological activity of the nervous system.

Signal	Reference	Source	BW[Hz]	BW_0[Hz]	Amp[μV]	Attribute
EEG	Lobes	Synapses	0-600	0-100	1-10	Osc Freq
EMG	Elbow	Motor unit	20-1000	20-400	100-1000	Power
EOG	Forehead	Retina-Cornea	0.05-35	0.05-10	500-1000	Rotation
ECG	Ankle	SA node	0.05-100	0.05-50	100-5000	Complex QRS
EDA		Sweet glands	0.045-0.25		0-5μ S	Trajectory

2.1.2 What is digital biosignal processing for?

Digital biosignal processing (DBP) is the mathematical manipulation of biosignals to obtain the greatest amount of information about the process that generates them (CNS and PNS). At present, one of the most prolific scientific areas (both at an academic and research level) is the DBP [379]. The growth of this area has been such that it has expanded to other sciences such as Neurosciences, Psychology, Therapies and Rehabilitation, Diagnostic Medicine, Mechatronics, Control and Automation, among others [498].

Unfortunately, teaching techniques for effective DBP learning have lagged behind. Frequently, students fail to understand, and obviously apply, basic concepts concerning the analysis of information in discrete time. For this reason, there is an urgent need to develop tools that allow instructors to efficiently illustrate the DBP process. This process can be undertaken in four main stages: (1) acquisition, (2) time analysis, (3) frequency analysis, and (4) time-frequency analysis. Along DBP principles, it is essential that students also understand the possible applications of this mathematical and computational analysis. For example, when the sense organs (sensors), the nervous system (connections) and/or effectors (actuators) of the human body are injured, individuals experience dysfunctions that affect the usual way they interact with their environment. These dysfunctions can be congenital, or acquired when suffering from an illness or after a trauma [20]. Some of the most common ways to reestablish the interaction of individuals with their environment, after the electrophysiological circuit has been interrupted, involve the use of drugs or surgical interventions. Another means to alleviate this social suffering refers to neuroengineering technology. For example, peripheral electrical activity is used to control prosthetics [254]. Furthermore, when persons suffer from a severe neuromuscular injury, they can become locked in their own body without being able to move any of their muscles. In these cases, technology is being developed to allow direct communication with the brain, that is, a brain-computer interface (BCI) [563]. The fundamental basis of all this neuroengineering technology is the processing and control of electrophysiological signals.

2.1.3 PhyGUI: A didactic tool to teach DBP

In light of the previous discussion, a MATLAB®-based computer application to illustrate DBP principles applied on electrophysiological signals is presented herein. This way, students cannot only understand DBP fundamentals but also may be able to apply them effectively. The general design of the PhyGUI application is organized in four tabs: (1) Data acquisition, (2) time-domain analysis, (3) frequency-domain analysis, and (4) time-frequency analysis.

2.1.3.1 Data acquisition

In this tab, the discretization of the following biosignals is illustrated: EEG, ECG, EMG, EOG, breathing and temperature. This tab depicts the acquisition pathway of biosignals: from the source (human body) to the acquired signal (discretized signal plotted on the lower axes). Users can choose among six different signals: neuronal, cardiac, muscular, respiratory, temperature and ocular. Signals were recorded by undergraduate students from the biomedical engineering stream at Tecnológico de Monterrey. On the x-axes, the association between time and samples is shown. The sampling frequency in each case is specified in the top right corner. See Figure 2.3.

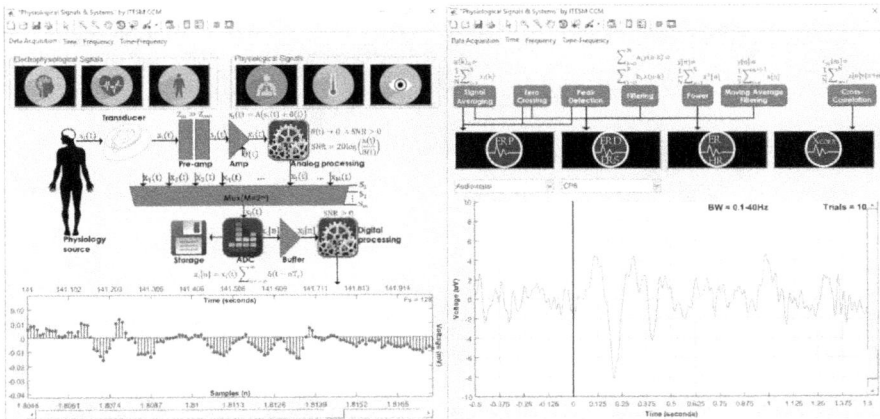

FIGURE 2.3: PhyGUI tabs: (1) discretization of biosignals on the left and (2) analysis on time domain on the right.

2.1.3.2 Time-domain analysis

Time-domain analysis can be encompassed under five categories: (1) average techniques, (2) zero crossing, (3) peak detection, (4) digital filtering and (5) power estimation. These strategies are commonly applied to estimate electrophysiological patterns such as event-related potentials (ERP), event-related (de-) synchronization (ERD/ERS) and event-related heart rate (ER-HR). To compare all these patterns, correlation and convolution are a great help. The integral application of the time-domain analysis strategies is presented in the tab 2 of the PhyGUI, as can be seen in Figure 2.3. In this tab, different event-related patterns can be explored and even compared (X_{corr}-button). The included events for neural responses (ERP and ERD/ERS) are auditory, visual and audiovisual. On the other hand, the included events for cardiac activity (ER-HR) are different levels of sensory-cognitive load.

2.1.3.3   Frequency-domain analysis

Frequency analysis is based on Fourier series (analysis and synthesis of biosignals) and Fourier transform (power spectral density and short-time Fourier transform). In tab 3 (Figure 2.4), the classical Fourier tools to analyze periodic signals (Fourier series) and non-periodic signals (Fourier transform) are shown. On the first axis, the sinusoidal components of an ECG signal are plotted with a dotted line. On the second axis, there is a demonstrative schematization of Parseval Theorem, which showed that the average energy in time is equal to the average energy in frequency. The signal presented on this axis is a respiratory signal recorded at 250 Hz. In addition, the respiratory spectrum is shown in orange. The average power value for time and frequency domains are respectively shown on the top left and right sides of the plot (Figure 2.4).

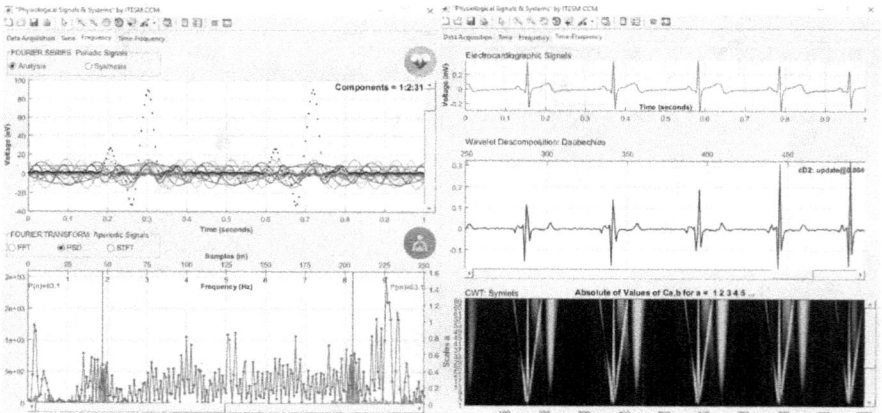

FIGURE 2.4: PhyGUI tabs: (3) frequency analysis based on Fourier series and transform on the left and (4) time-frequency based on Wavelet transform on the right.

2.1.3.4   Time-frequency analysis

The last tab refers to time-frequency analysis based on a Wavelet transform (Figure 2.4). Two main tools are included in the tab: (1) biosignal decomposition in time and (2) time-frequency analysis. On one hand, the decomposition of the ECG signal using the Daubechies Wavelet family can be explored in this tab. This strategy is very useful for implementing real-time systems, since it returns the frequency components at different response times. That is, the higher are the input signal frequencies, shorter is the response time. On the other hand, the scalogram estimated by applying continuous Wavelet transform (CWT) is depicted on the bottom axis of the tab. The CWT shows a good resolution plot in both domains of the ECG signal.

2.2 Analysis of electrophysiological activity

If an electrophysiological signal in the real world is defined as $x_e(t)$, then that signal must be discretized to study the electrophysiological mechanism into $x_e(t)$ by sampling the signal at a frequency known as F_s. As a result, $x_e(t)$ can be reconstructed via its discretized version defined as $x[n]$ for every nT_s value in accordance with

$$x[n] = x_e(t)|_{t=nT_s} \tag{2.4}$$

where $T_s = 1/F_s$ and n=...,-2,-1,0,1,2,...

2.2.1 Preprocessing of electrophysiological signals

As any other electrical phenomenon, electrophysiological signals are liable to the superposition of other electrical signals known as artifacts. In electrophysiology, artifacts can be categorized into: (1) exogenous, including environmental noise such as the line source, individual motion, high electrode impedance, electronic noise, and electrode-skin interface; and (2) endogenous that refers to any bioelectrical human information different to that under study. Therefore, the goal of signal preprocessing is to reduce the electrical activity superposed to the signal of interest. Namely, for the signal-to-noise ratio defined by Eq. 2.5 to tend to infinity, where P refers to the signal power.

$$SNR = \frac{P_{signal}}{P_{noise}} \to \infty \tag{2.5}$$

2.2.1.1 Referencing methods

The first step to reduce Pnoise is to reference the electrophysiological signals. These signals must be measured against a referencing point that ideally should be "inactive", electrically speaking. The referencing point depends on the biosignal at hand. In Table 2.1, common referencing sites for different biosignals are exemplified. This type of referencing method is known as monopolar since the differential potential measured is between an active electrode (r_i) and an inactive one (r_R). That is,

$$\phi(r_i,t) = V(r_i,r_R,t) \tag{2.6}$$

Monopolar referencing does not only reduce random and common signals (noise) merged into the biosignals, but also can modify the amplitude of ϕ. As a case in point, when a particular lobe is chosen as a reference, the EEG amplitude decreases on the electrodes that are close to the referencing electrode. When linked earlobes are chosen, the asymmetry effect of using one lobe referencing electrode is avoided. However, the link wire between two earlobe referencing electrodes affects intracranial currents that produce the EEG potentials. This inconvenient effect also produces a distortion on the EEG recording. Once the electrophysiological signals have been monopolarly referenced, they can be re-referenced by the bipolar referencing method that is defined as

$$\phi(r_{ij}, t) = V(r_i, r_R, t) - V(r_j, r_R, t) \tag{2.7}$$

where r_j refers to another active electrode differing from r_i.

In addition, EEG signals can be re-referenced by two additional methods: Laplacian and common average reference. In both cases, the methods proceed as follows

$$\phi(r_{ik}, t) = V(r_i, r_R, t) - \frac{1}{K} \sum_{k=1}^{K} V(r_k, r_R, t) \tag{2.8}$$

where k is the k-th electrode and K refers to the four (or eight) neighboring nearest electrodes to the i-th channel when the Laplacian referencing method is applied. In the case of the common average referencing method, K refers to the total number of EEG electrodes.

The referencing method determines the spatial filtering of the biosignals, which in turn maximizes the electrophysiological mechanisms of interest. This is why the selection of an optimal electrode montage, along with precise electrode location, is significant. For example, in [100], it was found that the best referencing electrode to discriminate between two motor imagery related tasks was FCz, a recording site localized over the supplementary motor area.

2.2.1.2   Signal conditioning

After referencing, the question that must be answered is: What is the bandwidth of my interest? Depending on the electrophysiological patterns under study, the bandwidth must be adjusted. For example, if essential information must be extracted, BW_0 (Table 2.1) is recommended. However, if the signals must be studied in detail, BW (Table 2.1) must be guaranteed. Two basic processing techniques to limit the bandwidth are available: (1) baseline correction and (2) digital filters. Baseline correction refers to removing the signal offset by

$$x'[n] = x[n] - \bar{x}[n] = x[n] - \frac{1}{N} \sum_{n=0}^{N-1} x[n] \tag{2.9}$$

Note that baseline correction is not only applied for signal conditioning, it is also a widely used technique to estimate neurophysiological changes, which are regularly detected with respect to baseline signals such as recordings at rest, or signal segments not influenced by physical or mental conditions of interest. Regarding digital filters, the most common type of filter used for Electrophysiology is the IIR Butterworth design [105]. Digital filters are maybe the most commonly used DBP tool. However, their use must be restricted since they frequently diminish the biosignal amplitude, an effect that is frequently overlooked.

2.2.1.3 Rejection and removal of artifacts

Physiological variability along the body is the main source of artifacts, depending on the electrophysiological signal features under study (such as magnitude and BW), electrode montage, and anatomy of the human body. For example, if EEG signals are under study, their main artifacts are eye movements including blinking (EOG), cardiac activity (ECG), and muscle activity (EMG). There are other influences such as respiration, tongue movements, tremor, and skin potentials, but these are far less frequent. EOG artefacts appear as high or low amplitude patterns in EEG recordings. These artefacts have a broad bandwidth, being maximal at frequencies below 4 Hz. As a consequence, they can be confused with delta and theta band rhythms. The strength of the EOG interference depends on the proximity of the electrodes to the eyes, and consequently, the EOG artefacts are much more prominent over the anterior recording sites. ECG and EMG are other common artifacts that interfere with the EEG signals. The ECG artifacts can cause a large interference depending on the user body shape and due to their wide frequency band (0.1–250 Hz). The EMG artefacts appear while contracting muscles such as when swallowing, frowning, chewing, or sucking. These artifacts range between 15 and 30 Hz, disturbing the beta band rhythms.

Visual Inspection can be seen as a tedious and outdated, or even unnecessary, stage. However, visual inspection allows the detection of transient artifacts including subject motion and bad electrodes. Bad electrodes refer to the transducers that inevitably move along the signal recordings, modifying the direct current potential at the electrode-skin interface. This causes abrupt changes in the baseline level of the recording. All these transient artifacts can be rejected manually or automatically. At present, there are efficient tools that automatically reject signal segments and/or bad electrodes. For example, Artifact Subspace Reconstruction is an available algorithm that undertakes artifact correction without causing serious signal loss [403]. Another example is the high-variance electrode artifact algorithm to remove transient electrode pop and drift artifacts [267].

Source Separation. Techniques for removing artifacts can be grouped in linear filtering and blind source separation. Linear filtering is useful when the they are well defined within frequency bands that do not overlap with those of the electrophysiological mechanism of interest. Blind source separation pursues to find the independent electrical sources that are generating the electrophysiological activity being recorded. As was aforementioned, physiological variability along the body is the main source of artifacts. As a result, the electrophysiological signals that are recorded (x) are the superposition of K different independent electrical sources (s). That is,

$$x = (x_1, x_2, \ldots, x_K) \tag{2.10}$$

$$s = (s_1, s_2, \ldots, s_K) \qquad (2.11)$$

$$x = \sum_{k=1}^{K} a_k s_k = AS \qquad (2.12)$$

Blind source separation methods aim to determine the independent electrical sources, and then, they remove unrelated sources and reconstruct signals without the undesired components. That is,

$$s = A^{-1}x = Wx \qquad (2.13)$$

where W is the contribution (weights) of each localized independent electrical source into the recording. The most applied method is Independent Component Analysis (ICA). ICA has been shown to be highly efficient to isolate the various source generating processes underlying electrophysiological recordings [240]. However, independent sources found by ICA decomposition must be manually inspected, selected, and interpreted, but doing so requires both time and practice. So far, there is a wide variety of tools to automatically assess and remove sources such as ICLabel [399], a tool that automatically identifies up to eight different sources: (1) neural, (2) muscular, (3) ocular, (4) cardiac, (5) line noise, (6) channel noise, and (7) others.

Electrode Interpolation aims to reconstruct bad electrodes by combining their neighboring electrodes on the basis that electrophysiological signals result from the superposition (Eq. 2.12) of the physiological activity generated across the human body. A useful tool to interpolate electrodes is PREP-pipeline [59].

2.2.2 Processing of electrophysiological signals

Electrophysiological signals can be processed in three domains: (1) time, (2) frequency, and (3) space. In each of these domains, the following aims are pursued:

- *Time* – To study the magnitude, morphology and topography of the signals.

- *Frequency* – To estimate the frequency composition of the signals.

- *Space* – To locate the electrical sources of the signals.

Time and frequency domains are the core of signal analysis. The essential tools to analyze the electrophysiological activity in each of these domains are described below.

2.2.2.1 Time Domain

Average Techniques. As noise is not correlated with the signal of interest, average techniques are applied to increase the signal-to-noise ratio in two ways: across time-windows and along the time-series. On one hand, whether several measurements of a signal are available, those trials can be averaged. Repeatable electrophysiological patterns will be augmented since they are being summed up, while random patterns as noise will be reduced. This technique is commonly used in quasi-periodic signals such as ECG, or in induced responses such as those obtained from EEG experimental paradigms. On the other hand, moving average filtering is another technique to reduce noise patterns applied along the time series. The filter order is higher whenever S is increased in Eq. 2.14. Note that if S is very high, the signal morphology can be affected.

$$y[n] = \frac{1}{S} \sum_{i=n}^{n+S-1} x[i] \qquad (2.14)$$

Zero Crossing and Peak Detection. The identification of the maximum value and/or the permutation between positive and negative magnitudes (and vice versa) into a time window are typical estimations to characterize the signal morphology. For example, it is common practice to detect the QRS complex of the ECG signal to estimate the heart rate variability that reflects the equilibrium between the sympathetic and parasympathetic nervous systems; zero crossings of EDA activity are frequently detected to monitor the metabolism of the human body, and peak values and zero crossings of breathing signals are generally identified to measure the level of energy consumption.

Power. Power refers to the amount of energy in a signal within a specific frequency bandwidth (absolute power), or even, against a particular frequency bandwidth (relative power). A typical feature of electrophysiological signals estimated is the mean band power, that is

$$y[n] = \frac{1}{N} \sum_{i=1}^{N} x_i^2[n] \qquad (2.15)$$

2.2.2.2 Frequency domain

The frequency content of a signal is essentially studied on the basis of Fourier series, in the case of periodic signals, and Fourier Transform, in the case of non-periodic signals. The first alternative is to analyze the frequency composition of a signal; namely, to estimate the weight that every frequency between 0 and $F_s/2$ has into the signal. That is,

$$X[m] = \sum_{n=0}^{N-1} x[n] e^{\frac{-2\pi jmn}{N}} \qquad (2.16)$$

It is important to have in mind that a discrete signal has a discrete spectrum and the relationship between time and frequency is in terms of N (total number of samples in time) and F_s (sample frequency) which is,

$$f_d = \frac{F_s}{N} \qquad (2.17)$$

where f_d refers to the frequency resolution. As a result, the recording length is directly associated with the spectrum resolution. The second alternative is to synthesize a signal, that is, to construct a signal by weighting and phasing a variety of sines and cosines.

2.2.2.3   Time-frequency domain

Time and frequency domains are related to each other by the Theorem of Plancherel. This theorem states that the accumulated power in time is equal to mean power in frequency, that is,

$$\sum_{n=0}^{N-1} x^2[n] = \frac{1}{N} \sum_{m=0}^{N-1} |X[m]|^2 \tag{2.18}$$

A method based on Fourier to analyze the spectrum changes along time is the Short-Time Fourier Transform. In this technique, the Fourier Transform is applied to time windows, and then, a time-frequency analysis is obtained. A drawback of this technique is to find the balance between time and frequency resolution. A way to find that balance is the Heisenberg's uncertainty principle:

$$\Delta f \Delta t \geq \frac{1}{4\pi} \tag{2.19}$$

2.2.3   Processing of EEG signals

Current standard models explain the existence of EEG signals but not their content. The main contributions have been coming from Cognitive Neurosciences (macroscopic investigation), Neurobiology (microscopic investigation), Mathematical Modelling, and Computational Analyses. Understanding the meaning of EEG may increase its usability to diagnose brain disorders, predict treatment outcome success, and increase the performance of EEG-based BCIs [104].

What is known up to now about EEG activity is reflects the functionality of CNS. EEG signals are the result of post-synaptic (excitatory and inhibitory) potentials coming from the pyramidal neural networks of the brain cortex. These neural networks locally and/or globally oscillate at specific frequencies to communicate with each other. Thus, the major EEG feature is the neural oscillations. These oscillations can be studied as they occur (spontaneous activity) without external influences, or elicited by sensory, emotional, cognitive and/or motor events (evoked and induced activity). Figure 2.5 outlines a wide variety of EEG signal processing techniques in the time, frequency, and space domains.

2.2.3.1   Spontaneous activity

As neural oscillations are the major EEG feature, the magnitude yielded by EEG activity within the well-known frequency bands ($\delta(0$–4 Hz), $\theta(4$–8 Hz), $\alpha(8$–12 Hz), $\beta(12$–30 Hz) and $\gamma(>30$ Hz)) is the main parameter of interest to be quantified. In the same line of thinking, the level of synchrony at specific frequency bands between two recording sites is also estimated. This EEG estimation is known as coherence and reflects the level of communication between neural networks. Coherence is the ratio of cross-power spectral density (S_{xy}), and power spectral densities of recording sites of interest (S_{xx} and S_{yy}), that is

$$Coh_{xy} = \frac{|S_{xy}(f)|^2}{S_{xx}(f)S_{yy}(f)} \qquad (2.20)$$

Linear methods as those abovementioned do not allow the study of the nature of EEG signals because neural oscillations are nonstationary, non-Gaussian and nonlinear. Recently, the concept of entropy has been included in EEG analysis since EEG signals are considered as a dynamic and stochastic system, which they are in reality. Some of the most commonly applied entropies in EEG analysis have been Shannon, Wavelet, Spectral and Hilbert-Huang [40]. For example, entropy has been applied (1) to understand and characterize different brain states and functions in healthy people [549], (2) to determine the level of functioning in individuals with autism [131], and (3) to investigate the emotional states using the minimum possible number of channels and frequency bands [344]. In addition, approximate entropy, along with its evolution (sample, multiscale, bivariate multiscale, and dynamic bivariate multiscale), has been widely applied by the scientific community. See Figure 2.5.

2.2.3.2 Evoked activity

Evoked activity refers to a transitory neural response due to sensory, perceptual, emotional, cognitive or motor events. This neural response is locked in time and phase. It is the result of the superposition of simultaneous postsynaptic potentials, and is commonly known as event-related potential (ERP).

The temporal properties of the ERPs are four: (1) polarity, (2) latency, (3) topographical distribution, and (4) sensitivity. Firstly, ERPs can be positive or negative peaks, and traditionally, their names are given in line with their polarity. Secondly, ERPs appear at a specific time after the event onset, and this latency is also used to name them. For example, the most common positive ERP appearing 300ms after an attentional event is known as P300. Finally, ERPs are found at specific recording sites depending on the event nature, which in turn, determines their sensitiveness. According to the previous example, P300 usually appears over frontal and occipital regions, which are highly associated with attentional mechanisms [310]. By way of illustration, Figure 2.6 presents auditory, visual and audiovisual ERPs across the whole scalp: from frontal up to occipital lobes. As can be seen from the figure, auditory ERPs appear over the frontal lobe where auditory information is interpreted, visual ERPs are brought about over the occipital lobe where visual stimulation is decoded, and audiovisual ERPs are a result of the integration of both previous neural transitory responses.

In addition to the analysis in the time domain, the identification of the frequency content of the ERPs, and the electrical sources where they are coming from is usually of interest. In terms of source localization, some of the most applied techniques are principal and independent component analyses.

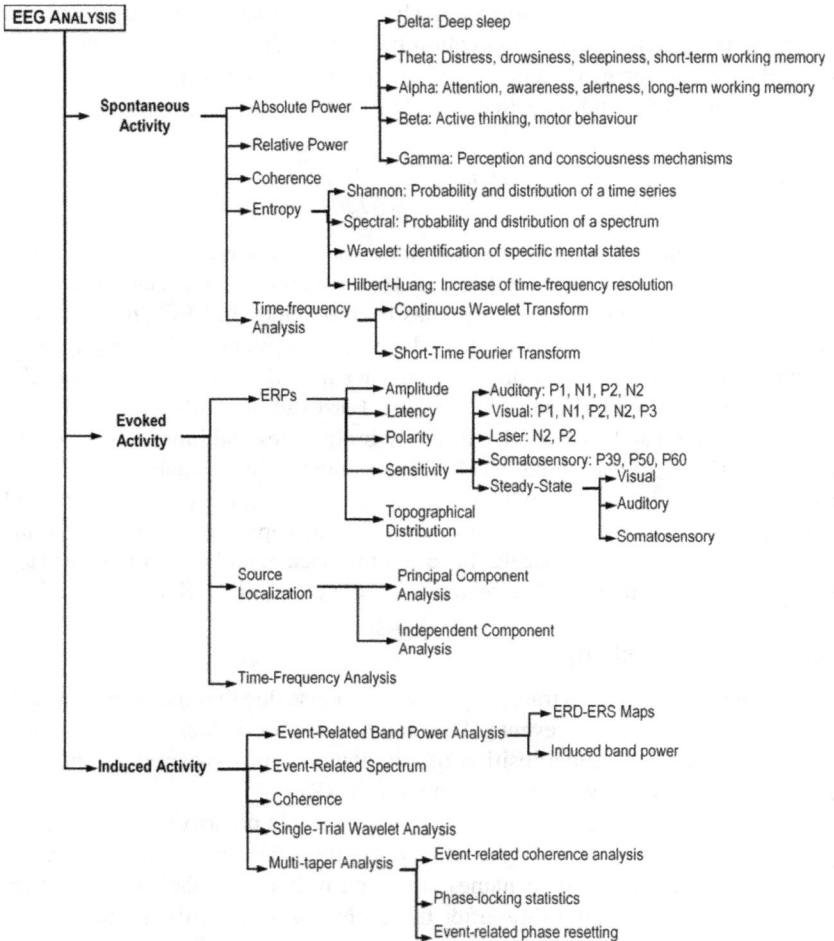

FIGURE 2.5: Outline of fundamental EEG signal processing techniques organized in spontaneous, evoked, and induced activity.

2.2.3.3   Induced activity

Induced activity refers to the quantification of the level of modulation of EEG signals induced by sensory, perceptual, emotional, cognitive or motor events. These event-related oscillations (EROs) are time-locked, but can or cannot be phase-locked. The synchronization of these EROs reflects a global coupling of the neural networks, that results in a signal power increase. In contrast, the desynchronization of EROs reflects local coupling, which in turn diminishes the signal power. EROs are very sensitive to frequency, and they are frequently estimated into narrow bands in the range, $2Hz \leq f \leq 6Hz$. When amplitude changes of EROs are of interest, event-

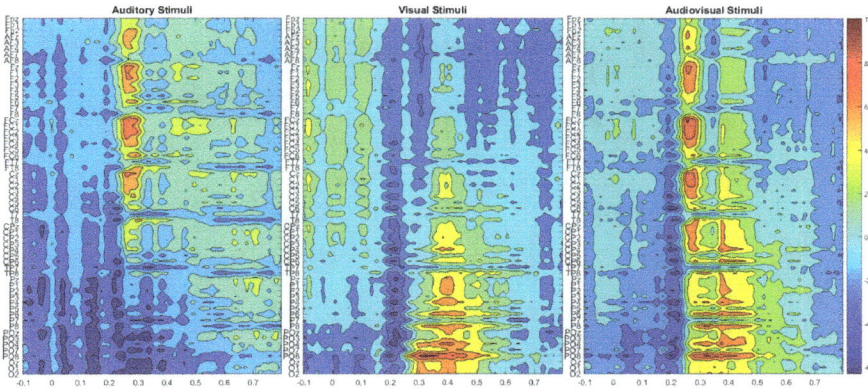

FIGURE 2.6: Auditory, visual and audiovisual ERPs. Auditory components are positive peaks appearing between 200 and 300 ms over prefrontal and frontal regions. Visual components are negative peaks around 200 ms, along with positive peaks between 300 and 400 ms, over the parieto-occipital region. Audiovisual components are the integrative effect of both stimulation modalities, auditory and visual.

related band power is estimated. When phase changes are under study, techniques including event-related phase resetting and coherence are taken into account.

In Figure 2.7, motor event related band power in seven bands is presented. The frequency bands refer to lower theta ($\theta_L = 4$–6 Hz), upper theta ($\theta_U = 6$–8 Hz), lower alpha ($\alpha_L = 8$–10 Hz), upper alpha ($\alpha_U = 10$–12 Hz), lower beta ($\beta_L = 16$–20 Hz), upper beta ($\beta_U = 20$–24 Hz), and gamma ($\gamma = 36$–42 Hz). The level of synchronization due to motor imagery activity of the left and right hands is being calculated over left (Figures 2.7A and 2.7C) and right (Figures 2.7B and 2.7D) sensorimotor regions of the brain cortex. As can be seen in the figure, motor imagery activity of the right hand elicits desynchronization into a majority of the bands over the contralateral hemisphere (Figure 2.7B). Contrary, synchronization of theta and alpha bands is present over the ipsilateral hemisphere. For left hand movements, EROs are not as clear as for the right hand. Since the individual was right-handed, this result was expected. Contralateral desynchronization along with ipsilateral synchronization over the sensorimotor cortex is a typical neural pattern associated with motor events. Motor mechanisms are commonly monitored by ERO mapping, as is illustrated in Figure 2.7.

2.2.4 Tools for electrophysiological analysis

So far, there are a wide variety of open-source softwares for processing electrophysiological signals. The most used toolboxes are EEGLAB, FieldTrip, BrainStorm and MNE, as can been in Figure 2.8. EEGLAB has become the leading tool for an electrophysiological activity because it is well-supported with up-to-date software that allows interaction in two ways: (1) graphical user interface and/or (2) line com-

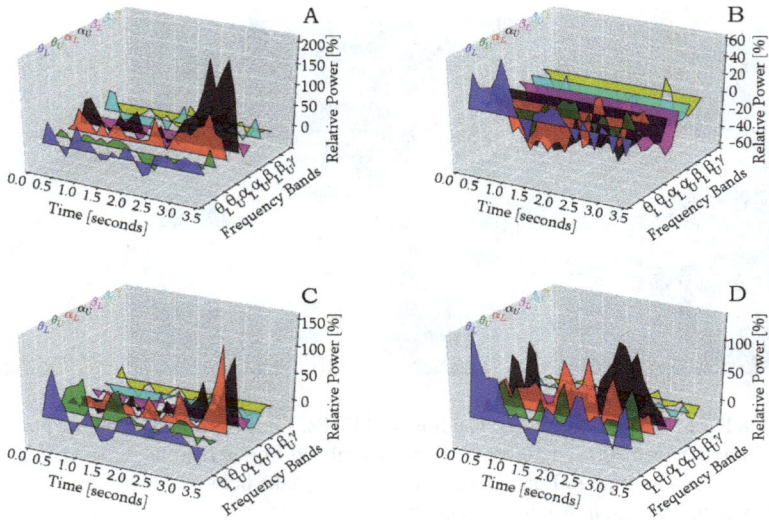

FIGURE 2.7: Motor event-related oscillations due to left and right hand opening. (A) EROs of left hand over left hemisphere. (B) EROs of right hand over left hemisphere. (C) EROs of left hand over right hemisphere. (D) EROs of right hand over right hemisphere.

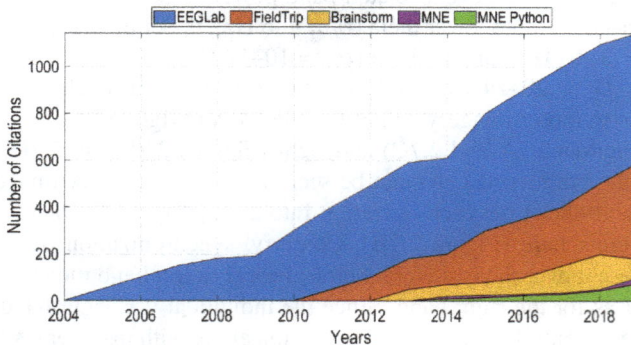

FIGURE 2.8: Usability tendencies of different platforms to analyze electrophysiological signals. EEGLAB implemented and maintained by the Swartz Center for Computational Neurosciences has been positioned as the major toolbox for electrophysiological analysis, in particular EEG signals [326].

mand [21]. In addition, the scientific community constantly contributes with plugins that increase EEGLAB functionality. All of the processing tools herein suggested are plug-ins for EEGLAB. FieldTrip is an open-source toolbox for MATLAB, as well. It was created by the Donders Institute of Brain for MEG and EEG analyses [326]. BrainStorm is an open-source application dedicated for analyzing MEG, EEG, fNIRS, ECoG, depth electrodes and multiunit electrophysiology [377]. Laslty, MNE is an open-source Python package for exploring, visualizing, and analyzing human neurophysiological data including, MEG, EEG, sEEG, ECoG, and NIRS [41].

It is important to move towards standard and transparent investigations, thus it is highly recommended to make use of already existing platforms that offer state-of-the-art processing techniques.

2.3   Neural engineering technology

Neural engineering is the technical and computational development to measure, analyze and manipulate neural information that can be measured in three ways (1) electric current, (2) magnetic fields and (3) oxygen consumption in order to establish communication with both CNS and PNS [386, 440]. So far, there are three types of neural technologies:

- Sensorial interfaces collect information from senses and drive sensorial data to the CNS. Visual and auditory neuro-prostheses are examples of sensorial interfaces.

- Motor interfaces read information from the CNS to effect motor actions. The most common examples are brain-computer interfaces and neuro-prostheses for upper and lower limbs.

- Cognitive interfaces aim to reestablish communication among neural networks.

The number of neural technology applications has been gradually increasing. The following five differing applications are discussed here under: (1) rehabilitation, (2) human performance, (3) evaluation of working environments, (4) user-centered design BCIs and (5) treatment monitoring.

2.3.1   Neuronal interface for the evaluation of mental rotation tasks

In patients that suffered from a cerebrovascular stroke that compromised motor related cortical areas, the process of rehabilitation tends to be harder than expected. Previous studies have linked mental rotation with motor planning and execution, but till date background studies that link mental rotation tasks with motor priming have not been found. In this study, two sample groups were analyzed (experimental and control). The experimental group performing mental rotation and motor tasks and the control group performing only motor tasks. ERD/ERS mean power were quantified for theta, alpha and beta frequency bands using EEGLAB from MATLAB and characteristics that define the behavior of the ERD/ERS were used to train a Linear Discriminant Analysis. A t-test was performed to evaluate the significant difference between the mean value of the experimental and the control group. The results showed that there was a significant difference in the mean power of the midline frontal theta band, for which it can be inferred that mental rotation tasks can play a role in motor priming.

2.3.2 EEG monitoring of vigil and fatigue states during Laparoscopic tasks

Fatigue decreases efficiency in performance of several professional activities; therefore, being in that state could trigger technical mistakes whose consequences could be lethal, such as in the health area, where a surgical error due to the absence of rest can lead to patient death. For this reason, in this study the vigil and fatigue (due to sleep) states, that affect cognitive processes in medical students, were identified through EEG patterns. The EEG signals of 18 physician students were analyzed within θ band (4–8 Hz) over fronto-central recording sites, and α band (8–13 Hz) rhythms over temporal and parieto-occipital recording sites during the execution of laparoscopic tasks before and after their guard. The signal-processing pipeline consisted in preprocessing based on individual component analysis, absolute band power estimates, and Support Vector Machine classification. The f-score to differ between vigil and fatigue was 90.89%, where the first state showed more slightly identifiable EEG patterns reaching a sensitivity of 90.18%.

2.3.3 Environmental noise at library learning commons affects electrophysiological functioning

Environmental noise is an important social issue that directly affects the efficiency of the students. The aim of this study is to investigate how environmental noise affects the performance at leaning commons, a common novelty in education. For this study, sixteen students of Tecnológico de Monterrey (Nuevo León, México) were recruited: nine men and seven women (ages between 18 and 25). They were divided into four groups, and two collaborative activities were undertaken: (1) to solve a puzzle of 300 pieces without noise, and (2) to solve another puzzle of 300 pieces with noise at 75-80 dBA (same environmental noise found in leaning commons at Tecnológico de Monterrey). In both scenarios, the performance and the physiological reaction of students were investigated by (1) a summative evaluation based on the level of puzzle completeness, and (2) the electrophysiological monitoring of heart and blink rate, and neural electrical activity. The findings of the present study suggest that collaborative work is difficult to undertake in learning commons, when no appropriated policies are established and followed. Student performance was 4% higher in a quiet room than in learning commons. Noise in learning commons increased heart and blink rates by 3.48% and 22.91% respectively, regardless of task demands. Mental resources were reduced at least by 3% due to the environmental noise. As a result, cognitive performance when doing collaborative tasks at hand is lower than in quiet conditions. The level of noise at learning commons in Tecnológico de Monterrey could moreover increase readiness to react aggressively to everyday life situations in students.

2.3.4   Do user-centered designed paradigms for BCIs improve the modulation of EEG signals?

The aim of this project was to compare the level of modulation of the EEG activity achieved by 18 users under two paradigms: traditional (or Graz) and User-Centered Design (UCD). Both approaches made use of the same motor task: imagination of throwing out a basketball into a basket. The task was performed during online brain-computer communication. To quantify and qualify the level of modulation of the EEG signals, Wavelet entropy was applied since it is a nonlinear parameter that reveals the nature of EEG signals such as dynamic and non-stationarity of neurophysiological mechanisms, in contrast to commonly used lineal methods. Results showed that UCD approaches improve the modulation of EEG signals by providing more attractive, efficient, stimulating and novel experiences; and the average performance increased from 52.7±0.028% (traditional paradigm) to 60.1±0.005% (UCD paradigm). The performance was almost 10% higher in UCD than in traditional approaches, despite the fact that users posed the same motor imagery skills in line with the Motor Imagery Questionnaire.

2.3.5   How effective are acoustic therapies for tinnitus? A psychometric and neurophysiological evaluation

At present, a majority of the top tinnitus treatments is based on sound. Sound-based therapies may become highly effective when the right patient at the right time in the appropriate context is selected. The investigation presented here attempts to compare sound therapies based on music, retraining, neuro-modulation, and binaural sounds in line with (1) neuro-audiology assessments and (2) psychological evaluations. Sound-based therapies were tested in 76 patients with chronic and refractory tinnitus for two months. The neuro-audiology assessment was based on the estimation of the approximate entropy of the electrical neural activity. This assessment revealed that the whole frequency structure of the neural networks showed a higher level of activeness in tinnitus sufferers than in control individuals. Then psychological evaluation showed that retraining treatment tended to be the most effective sound-based therapy to reduce tinnitus perception, but it may be not recommended for individuals with anxiety. Binaural sounds and neuro-modulation produced very similar effects at reducing tinnitus perception, stress and anxiety. Music therapies should be recommended with caution since they may worsen tinnitus conditions due to their frequency content.

3

Applications of Machine Learning Classifiers in Epileptic Seizure Detection

Mohammad Kubeb Siddiqui and *Ruben Morales-Menendez**

3.1 Introduction

It is necessary to start with a detailed description of epilepsy, seizures, types of seizures, why seizures originate, the phases of the attack, methods to control seizures, and locating the affected lobes of the brain. This information allows us to understand the basic concepts of the neurological disorder and establishes its results and outcomes.

The word 'Seizure' is very relevant in epilepsy. This can be defined as a situation wherein communication between brain cells excites or inhibits other brain cells, and an imbalance is created in brain neurons, causing some chemical changes and electron surges this causes seizures, [214]. A seizure is a sudden collapse of neuronal activity in the brain that impulsively causes an involuntary alteration in behavior, sensation, and momentary loss of consciousness, usually lasting a few seconds or a few minutes. Seizures can happen to a person at any time and during any activity (such as driving, walking, talking, and swimming), leading to severe injuries: fractures and burns, which also result in death [55].

A single seizure is not considered a disease, but when more than one recurrent seizure with symptoms occurs, it is called epilepsy. It is a kind of chronic neurological disorder that affects more than 70 million people around the world. The word epilepsy is derived from a Latin word meaning *seizure* and has been known for more than 3,000 years; the *Babylonians* observed it and mentioned it in their medical text [432]. Epilepsy has spread to all mammalian species [165], and many pharmaceutical researchers have tested *AntiEpileptic Drugs* (*AED*) in rats and mammalian species [278]. The word epilepsy does not indicate anything about the cause or severity of the seizures. It has been distributed evenly and without complications throughout the world. The Figure 3.1 presents a general idea of seizure and non-seizure from the *EEG* signals.

There are several theories about the causes of seizures. Seizures occur due to a disturbance in the electrical activity of the brain; has genetic factors that induce

---

School of Engineering and Sciences, Tecnologico de Monterrey, Monterrey, Mexico.
* Corresponding author: rmm@tec.mx

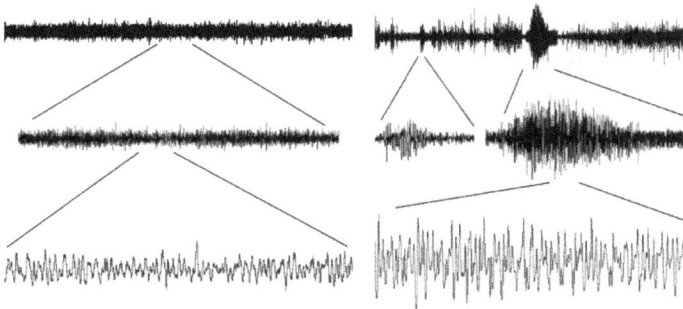

FIGURE 3.1: Non-seizure spikes (left) and Seizure (right).

several other irregularities [412, 475] such as brain malformations, lack of oxygen during delivery, low blood sugar, blood calcium, blood magnesium, or other electrolyte disturbances, inborn metabolism errors, intracranial hemorrhage, maternal drug, febrile seizures, brain tumor in rare cases, brain infections, congenital conditions (*Down* syndrome; *Angelman* syndrome; tuberous sclerosis and neurofibromatosis), progressive brain disease (rare), head trauma, cerebrovascular incident, some cases of epilepsy, but it can also be the result of brain injury, stroke, infection, high fever or tumors [352, 452]. The occurrences of epilepsy are not conditioned by limits such as racial, geographic or social, gender, and age, but its incidence is more in childhood and in the elderly [412]. World-renowned personalities such as *Nobel* prize winners, olympic medalists, and philosophers who have had epilepsy still gained recognition in their respective fields.

Epilepsy remains a reflective community problem due to ingrained historical concepts of supernatural or sacred disorders; ignorance, fear, misunderstandings, and humiliation contributed to severe and incurable outcomes in this disease. Fortunately, several organizations were born to raise awareness and improve treatment, including the *International League Against Epilepsy* and the *International Office of Epilepsy*, affiliated to the *WHO* [169, 432].

3.1.1   Impact of epilepsy

There are some severe consequences of epilepsy; the patient suffers from the daily lifestyle unmanageabilities [488]:

- *I'm not doing well* at home, school, work, or with friends.

- Learning or cognitive problems that require specialized help or accommodations.

- Symptoms of depression, anxiety, or other changes in mood or behavior.

- Trouble sleeping.

- Injuries, falls, or other unexplained illnesses.

- Thinning of the bones or osteoporosis.

- Reproductive problems.

- Risk of death.

Around 40% of epileptic patients have no identification of their seizures. This percentage decreases with the help of *EEG* and *MRI* [431]. Still, it would help if more attention was paid to applying data mining techniques. Treating epilepsy is a challenge in itself; *AED* can treat it in some patients. In other cases, it is managed by surgical removal of an epileptic portion of the brain, and in others, it is difficult to treat due to its inappropriate nature. This shows that the importance given to research on epileptic seizure topics is quite impressive. The study shows that most epileptic patients have no causes of seizures [127, 452]. However, the roots of seizures are identified by different seizure control devices, such as *EEG*. Detecting epileptic seizures is in itself a critical challenge; approximately 70% of epileptic patients can be controlled with *AED*, if properly treated.

It has been observed that patients must take medications throughout their lives (this is for cases of tonic-clonic seizures). Others can be treated by surgically removing an epileptic portion of the brain. Finally, others are difficult to handle due to their nature. It is imperative to detect epileptic seizures using *ML* methods.

3.1.2 Phases of seizure

In epileptic seizures, the term *ictal* also comes in the literature. It also means a seizure. The seizure has four main stages [99, 166, 536]:

Pre-ictal means the time before the seizure. It can be seconds, minutes or days. The stage is not the same for every patient; it applies to those who do experience this stage. Not every patient experiences something different at this stage of a seizure; some of them who experience a *pre-ictal* stage, use it as an alert to prepare for the seizure or a safe place [536].

Ictal means seizure. There will be changes in the patient's body; the electrical storm in the patient's brain comes to life. During this stage, an alteration found in cardiovascular metabolism and changes in the *EEG* signals can be noted, [153].

Inter-ictal explains the time that elapses between seizures, [170, 496]. More than 50% of epileptic patients suffer from temporal lobe epilepsy; these result in emotional disturbances between seizures, including anxiety and depression.

Post-ictal means post-attack stage [144]. The stage counts from minutes to an hour. It depends on the type, intensity, and duration of the seizure. Activities vary from person to person, and patients may experience various disorders, such as headache, vomiting, confusion, and loss of consciousness. In most cases, patients do not remember what happened to them during a seizure [270].

3.1.3   Seizure types

People can experience an epileptic seizure and its different versions. The neuro-experts divided seizures into two categories, as shown in Table 3.1, *Partial Seizure*, which affects one section of the brain, and *Generalized Seizure*, which affects the entire brain [166, 495].

TABLE 3.1: Main types of seizures.

Partial Seizure	Simple partial seizure Complex partial seizure
Generalized Seizure	Generalized convulsive seizure Generalized non-convulsive seizure

3.1.3.1   Partial seizure

In partial seizure, a particular region of the brain or a set of brain cells is affected; therefore, it is also called a *focal seizure* [495, 170]. When only a region in one side of the brain is affected, abnormal activities start in it. Further, it moves to another, or it just positions itself in a single area. Partial seizures affect the functioning of related human body organs, e.g., if occipitalis is involved, then the human speaking ability also gets affected. When the patient suffers from this type of seizure attack in that moment the patient is aware of the surroundings and keeps consciousness level is retained. Further, a partial seizure is classified into two subcategories: *simple partial* and *complex partial* seizure.

Simple partial: Patients are aware of their surroundings, but cannot consciously perform any activity, such as talking until the seizure passes. Typical symptoms are that the patient rolls his/her eyes, shakes himself/herself, shakes his/her hands and feet. The seizure affects a different part of the brain; instead, the emotions of the patient or senses may be affected [495].

Complex partial: It does not focus on a specific region of the brain, but affects multiple parts. It also affect the level of consciousness. Although, complex partial seizures can affect any region of the brain, they usually occur in one area of the two temporal lobes of the brain. Due to this nature, people are prone to complex partial seizures and are often called *Temporal Lobe Epilepsy (TLE)*. Above all, it affects one of the temporal lobes of the brain. The main symptoms are chewing, snapping fingers, pinching clothing, walking for no reason, and mumbling. The patient experiences confusion lasting several minutes after the seizure [383].

3.1.3.2   Generalized seizure

Abnormal activities affect the entire region of the brain, and the patient loses consciousness. There are two types: generalized convulsive and generalized non-convulsive, [164].

- Generalized convulsive seizures

  They include four types of seizures - myoclonic, clonic, tonic, and tonic-clonic.

  Myoclonic seizure: A segment of the patient's body suddenly contracts. The name *Myoclonus* is a *Greek word* meaning muscle, and *klonus* refers to confusion, because this is where muscle contraction and relaxation occur [551].

  Clonic seizure: *Clonus* (KLOH-nus) refers to muscle contraction and relaxation in a rapid manner or repeated jerks. It is very similar to myoclonic, but contraction and relaxation are slower. It can be diagnosed at any age, from infancy to old age. The movements cannot be stopped by restricting or repositioning the arms or legs [5].

  Tonic seizure: Patients' muscles stiffen while the seizure occurs. This random contraction of the trunk and face muscles is accompanied by stretching, and the patient maintains [5, 455] consciousness. It occurs mainly during sleeping hours, and in this, all or most of the brain is affected. The duration of these seizures is less than 20 seconds. After this seizure, the patient may or may not be dizzy or confused.

  Tonic-clonic seizure: It is known as *grand mal epilepsy* [205]. Both electrographic and clinical events simultaneously involved bilateral brain networks. The parts of the patient's body begin to shake uncontrollably. During this time, your tongue is bitten by the teeth, shortness of breath occurs, among other effects. The patient feels confused for a short time facing problems identifying friends and family. After the seizure, the patient feels a headache, vomits, and needs deep sleep. The tonic-clonic seizure lasts between one and two minutes, but the patient may not regain consciousness for 10 to 15 minutes [205].

- Generalized non-convulsive seizures

  They are of two main types, absence and atonic seizures.

  Absence seizure: In its absence, the seizure patient suffers from a sudden onset of seizures without any aura; it begins and ends abruptly; also, there is a momentary loss of consciousness. This frequency of seizures is much higher than what can be repeated more than once a day; its duration, also lasts a few seconds [321]. It can be controlled by *AED*. It is more common in children than in adults.

  Atonic seizure: It is known by different names, such as *a gout attack* or *static* or *akinetic seizure*. It is very unpredictable and has severe consequences, and traumatic injuries [541]. These seizures cause some or all aspects of the body to weaken suddenly; the patient does not lose consciousness. Then the patient's head suddenly falls and collapses, falling to the ground. People are victims of this seizure, and a doctor advises them to wear caps [352].

3.1.4 Lobes of brain

The brain regions are shown in Figure 3.2; the cerebral cortex is the largest part of the human brain, associated with higher brain functions, such as thinking and action. The cerebral cortex is divided into four sections, called lobes [341, 462, 491, 562]. The Frontal lobe, the Parietal lobe, the Occipital lobe, and the Temporal lobe [9]. The description of various lobes is presented in Table 3.2.

TABLE 3.2: Specific jobs of each lobe.

Brain lobe	Association
Frontal (F)	reasoning, planning, parts of speech, movement, emotions, and problem-solving
Parietal (P)	training, orientation, recognition, perception of stimuli
Occipital (O)	visual processing
Temporal (T)	perception and recognition of auditory stimuli, memory, and speech

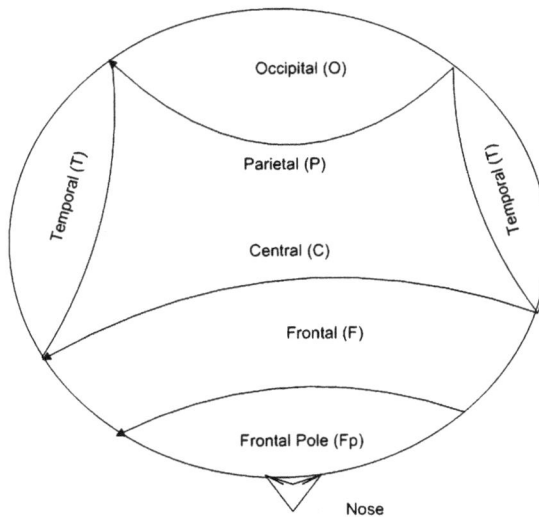

FIGURE 3.2: Brain lobes.

3.2 Epileptic seizure monitoring tool

The background and significance of monitoring electrical brain signals are discussed, such as, technical descriptions of these devices.

3.2.1 Electroencephalography

German psychiatrist Hans Berger, [53], from the University of Jena, Germany, first recorded electrical signals from the human brain using an *EEG* in 1921, [185]. Hans Berger's first publication was based on the human *EEG* in 1929; revealing that continuous and regular potential changes could be recorded each time a sensitive string galvanometer was connected to a subject's head in a relaxed supine position via suitable electrodes [53, 216]. Canadian neuroscientist Dr. Herbert H. Jasper studied the *EEG* tool's mechanisms and applied it to record the electrical signals of neurons responsible for different brain activities in the states of consciousness, learning, and epileptic electron discharge [351, 428, 236]. Dr. Jasper collaborated with Canadian neurophysiologist Wilder Penfield, who revolutionized *EEG* in epilepsy.

EEG of a non-invasive scalp method of capturing electrical signals from the brain through electrodes/channels implanted on the surface of a person's skull is a painless technique. *EEG* signal traces show differences between potential electrodes. The possible differences are due to the communication between neurons that send and receive electrical signals. Each neuron contributes to the tracking of the small activities by *EEG*. The *EEG* will pick up a signal only when a group of neurons explodes simultaneously; this signal is amplified to give us the best reading. The *EEG* cannot be used to tell what someone is thinking. However, it can provide us with information about human emotions, such as thinking, fear, anger, sleep, joy, and wakefulness.

EEG is widely used to diagnose neurological disorders, including epilepsy. Epilepsy is one of the most common neurological diseases, and in this, the *EEG* is very demanding to evaluate the brain signals of epileptic patients [151, 367]. *EEG* signals visualize the different patterns of electrical activity in the brain (normal, abnormal).

Some abnormal *EEG* signal patterns can occur due to various unfavorable conditions, for example, seizures, strokes and head trauma. An example of this is known as *slowing*; the brain waves are slower; we await the patient's level of alertness and age. Not only for epilepsy, but it is also useful for diagnosing other neurological disorders such as dementia and *Alzheimer*. It spontaneously records the electrical activities generated in the cerebral cortex. Typically, *EEG* signals are involved, chaotic, with non-linear dynamic properties, long-duration, and time-varying recordings, and produce a large volume of data.

The *EEG* is one of the tools to diagnose epileptic seizures, analyzing the different behaviors of brain signals, and providing *ictal* and *interictal* activities. An example of an *EEG* is shown in Figure 3.3, where the *x-axis* is the number of samples (time) and the *y-axis* is the amplitude in μV. The main contribution is that it classifies the different types: normal when displaying distinct signal patterns such as sharp peaks, flattened, etc., [94]. If a patient has partial seizures, the sharp spikes and waves on the *EEG* in a particular area of the brain, such as the temporal lobe, can recognize where the seizures originate. The *EEG* helps identify different brain signal patterns, classifies them into epileptic seizures and other paroxysmal non-epileptic seizures [365, 524]. It also helps to identify the types of seizures, as shown in Figure 3.4 with the following patterns: sharp waves, spikes, benign epileptiform discharges of

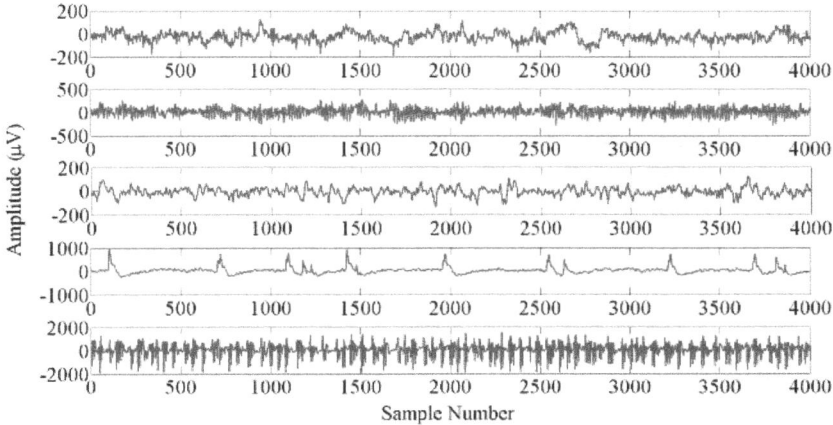

FIGURE 3.3: Sample of *EEG* signals captured from different implanted electrodes.

childhood, wave complexes, spike-wave complexes, spike-wave complexes, seizure pattern and polyspikes.

ElectroencephaloGram

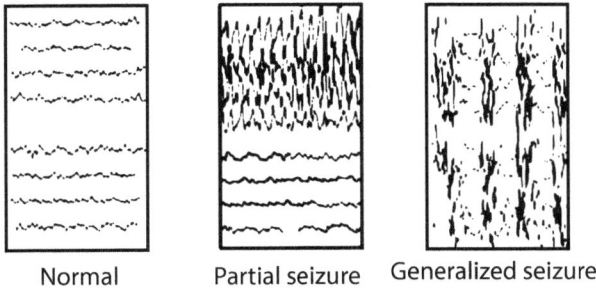

Normal   Partial seizure   Generalized seizure

FIGURE 3.4: *EEG* signal shows different types of epileptic seizures.

3.2.1.1   10–20 international system

These recordings are made using electrodes implanted on the surface of the brain in a non-invasive way. Electrode implantation follows the International System 10–20 standard, [282]. This standard describes the electrodes' location on the scalp; it is based on the relationship between the implanted electrode and the region of the cerebral cortex. The purpose of writing 10–20 indicates the distances between the adjacent electrodes, which are 10% or 20% of the entire right to the left and from the front to the back of the scalp. To place the electrodes there, four anatomical locations are required: nasion, inion, and left/right preauricular points. The nasion is located between the forehead and the nose, and inion is located at the lowest point of the scalp located at the bottom of the external occipital protrusion [250, 526].

The even series of electrodes is implanted in the right region of the cerebral hemisphere. The odd series of electrodes are placed in the left area of the cerebral hemisphere. Figure 3.6 shows the percentage of distances between the electrodes; each electrode is connected to its adjacent electrode in a specific gap such as 10%, 20%, and 25%. The implantation of electrodes in the *International 10–20 System* representing all electrode pairs such as 6, 48, 44, and 12 are implanted on the scalp's right side. Instead, a strange series of electrodes like 3, 19, 43, and 61 are placed on the scalp's left side. Each number defines the scalp location of lobes (**F**rontal, **T**emporal, **P**arietal, **C**entral and **O**ccipital.)

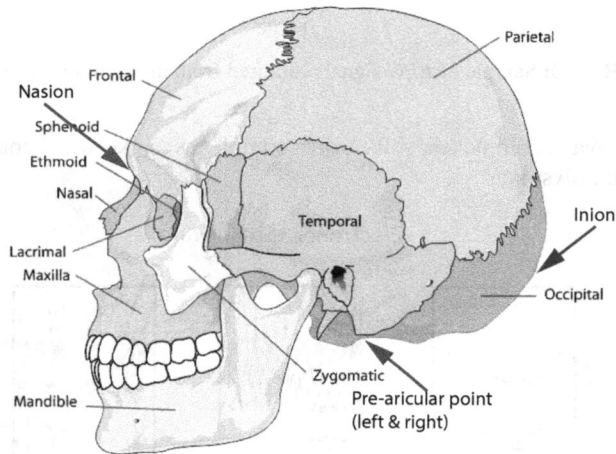

FIGURE 3.5: Anatomical landmarks for the positioning of electrodes (Adapted from [350]).

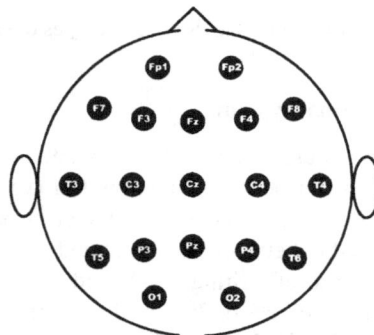

FIGURE 3.6: Distance of electrodes on the scalp as per 10–20 System [467].

Hardware Configuration:

64 Channel EEG

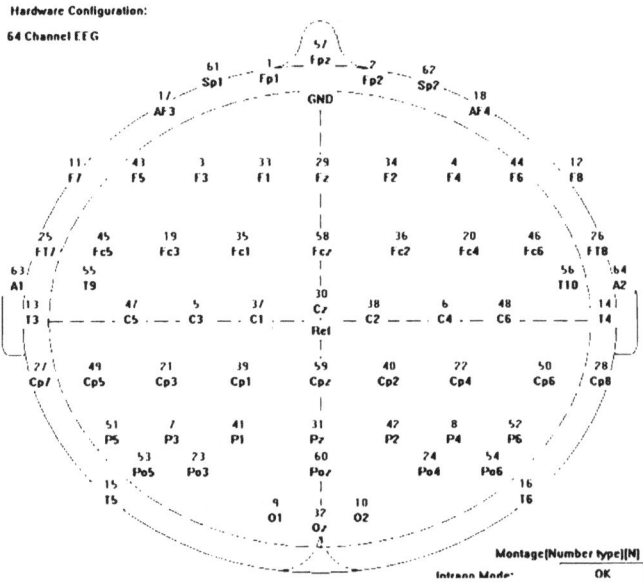

FIGURE 3.7: Implantation of electrodes on the scalp as per 10–20 System [467].

3.2.2   Electrocorticography

ECoG is a method to record electrical activity that occurs in the brain. The electrodes are directly on the cerebral cortex; they are small in size and are made of silver, platinum, or stainless steel embedded at a distance of 10–15 mm in soft and flexible silicone plastic strips with 8–16 contacts [488]. It has an important relationship with detecting epileptic seizures; the significant difference between *EEG* and *ECoG* is that the latter is an invasive system. The difference between *EEG* and *ECoG* implantation can be seen in Figure 3.9.

ECoG signals are preferred because they provide better *SNR* (*signal-to-noise ratio*). Invasive electrodes are implanted subdurally in the grid-like cortex or stereotactically placed in functional brain tissue (parenchyma), Figure 3.8 [366, 367]. The invasive form did not provide any physical pain to the patient [283]. An investigation by M. Kramar [273] has used the data set *ECoG*; In this, there are 76 electrodes implanted in the scalp, of which a grid of 12 electrodes is invasively planted. The remaining 64 electrodes are implanted on the surface of the scalp in a non-invasive method.

The main importance of applying the *ECoG* monitoring method is that it provides temporal and spatial images with high resolution [518] and a pattern of different peaks [388]. *ECoG* is performed before presurgical Epilepsy evaluation, which generally considers scalp recordings via *EEG*. This facilitates surgical operations for brain injuries.

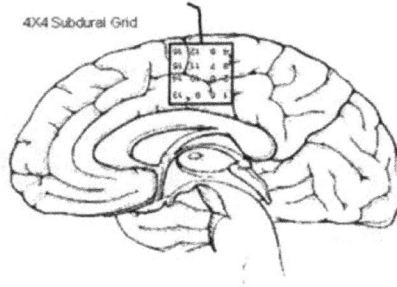

FIGURE 3.8: A grid of electrodes implanted in an invasive manner.

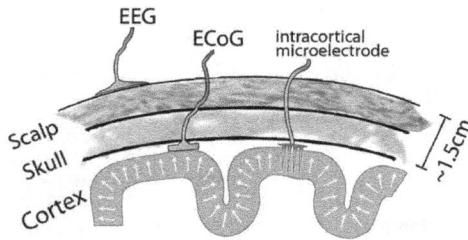

FIGURE 3.9: Implantation of invasive (*ECoG*) and Non-invasive (*EEG*) electrodes.

3.3   Machine learning methods

As a data scientist, before applying *ML* techniques to real-world datasets, it is necessary to understand these techniques and their use.

ML is an important part of *Artificial Intelligence* (*AI*); plays a crucial role in the development of human interactive models. *ML* classifiers use statistical programs and techniques to reveal the patterns of large sets of raw data. These sensible logic patterns are used to make predictions on invisible data with a higher rate of precision. There is no standard definition of *ML*, but different organizations and universities have provided its meaning.

1. "*ML* is the science of getting computers to act without being explicitly programmed." – Stanford.

2. "*ML* algorithms can figure out how to perform important tasks by generalizing from examples." – University of Washington.

3. "The field of *ML* seeks to answer the question, "How can we build computer systems that automatically improve with experience, and what are the fundamental laws that govern all learning processes?" – Carnegie Mellon University.

4. "*ML*, at its most basic, is the practice of using algorithms to parse data, learn from it, and then decide or predict about something in the world." – Nvidia.

5. "*ML* is based on algorithms that can learn from data without relying on rules-based programming."- McKinsey & Co.

ML has been in high demand as it can solve and improve real-world problems, such as, disease diagnosis, cybersecurity and consumer behavior [4, 6, 19, 139, 484, 387, 483]. After getting the dataset from *EEG* signals, *ML* methods are applied. *ML* methods are of three types: *Supervised Learning Methods* (*SLM*), *Unsupervised Learning Methods* (*ULM*) and *Reinforcement Learning Methods*. While reinforcement learning is used in robotics, gaming and navigation areas, the SLM and ULM are used for classification problems.

3.3.1   Supervised learning methods

It is a kind of *ML* method, that plays an important role in discovering meaningful patterns from data sets from different domains. The dataset has non-class attributes and a predefined class attribute. It finds the relationship between non-class attributes and class attributes, also called target attributes, which accurately predict each case's target attribute in the dataset. The nature of the class attribute is discrete, for example, seizure, no seizure, or 0.1 [22, 272]. Table 3.3 shows the values obtained from the *EEG* signals; the non-class (A) attributes are C_1, C_2, C_3, and C_4. The class attribute (C) has two class values: *ictal* and *pre-ictal*. Popular *SLMs* are: *Decision tree*, *Decision Forest* (set of decision trees), *Support Vector Machine* (*SVM*), *K-Nearest Neighbors* (*KNN*), *Artificial Neural Networks* (*ANN*), etc.

TABLE 3.3: Sample of *EEG* signals values showing class/non-class attributes.

Channel-1	Channel-2	Channel-3	Channel-4	Class Attribute
134.22	0.29	1322.23	4.11	Ictal
143.11	0.19	1422.85	2.99	Ictal
351.05	0.84	1978.76	1.79	Ictal
195.02	1.15	1975.03	3.31	Pre-Ictal
174.01	0.75	992.69	7.01	Pre-Ictal
114.20	0.46	355.56	1.12	Pre-Ictal
351.05	0.84	1970.76	1.79	Ictal
195.02	1.15	1975.03	3.31	Pre-Ictal
174.01	0.75	992.69	7.01	Pre-Ictal
195.02	1.15	1975.03	3.31	Pre-Ictal
174.01	0.75	992.69	7.01	Pre-Ictal
114.20	0.46	355.56	1.12	Pre-Ictal
351.05	0.84	1978.76	1.79	Ictal
195.02	1.15	1975.03	3.31	Pre-Ictal

3.3.1.1   Decision tree

A *Decision Tree* is a logic-based *SLM*. Its basic structure consists of three main parts: nodes, leaves, and lines. The lines create connections between nodes and leaves. Rectangular and oval shapes represent nodes and leaves, respectively [207]. The *Decision Tree* has different levels (e.g., level 0, level 1, level 2, etc.); the top level is a root node, as shown in Figure 3.10. To build the *Decision Tree*, different impurity measures are used, such as *Information Gain*, *Gini Index*, and *Gain Ratio*, based on the attribute being selected with a root node representing a division point where it divides the quality of partition in a data set [414, 311].

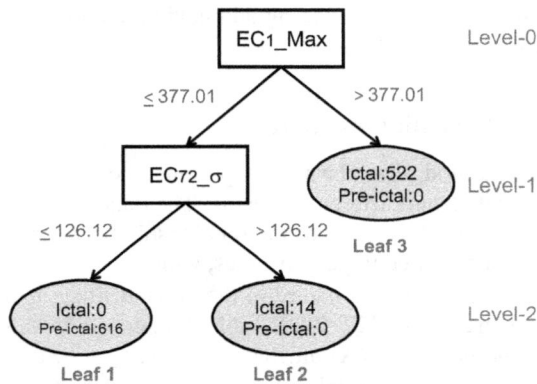

FIGURE 3.10: A Decision Tree used for *ictal* (seizure) and *pre-ictal* (pre-seizure) states.

Quilan used *Information Gain* to create decision trees, [414]. *Information Gain* is used for selecting the most potential attribute among the non-class features.

$$E(D) = -\sum P(CA_i, D) * (log_2(P(CA_i, D))) \qquad (3.1)$$

Equation (3.1) represents the Entropy of a dataset D, where CA is the class attribute and P is the probability of the class attribute over the dataset.

$$E(A_i, D) = -\sum D_i D * E(D_i) \qquad (3.2)$$

The dataset has been split into a segment, and the entropy of each component has been calculated by equation (3.2). The *Information Gain* of the dataset is calculated by equation (3.3):

$$E(A_i, D) = E(D) - E(A_i, D) \qquad (3.3)$$

3.3.1.2   Decision forest

Decision Forest is a *non-black-box* classification technique. It is a group of multiple diverse *Decision Trees* [73]. Each *Decision Tree* provides various logic rules, and probably different accuracy [160]. The *Decision Tree* of a *Decision Forest* behaves as a base classifier applied to classify the records as grouping behavior. Due to this nature, they are known as *ensemble* learning methods. The main objective of building the *Decision Forest* is that sometimes a single *Decision Tree* may be a *week learner*. When these *Decision Trees* get to come into a group format of *Decision Trees*, they become a *strong learner*. They are quite helpful in the knowledge discovery process [11]. In seizure detection, by analyzing several classifiers, it has been noted that the *Decision Forest* approach is more capable [479].

3.3.1.3 Random forest

A *Decision Forest* overcomes some of the disadvantages of a *Decision Tree*. In the *Decision Tree*, only a single set of logical rules can be discovered. The logical rules found by a single *Decision Tree* may fail to predict and classify class values correctly. *Random Forest* is a set of correlated *Decision Trees* and multiple *Decision Trees*, Figure 3.11. It is used to order any subset of data (instance) using a majority vote [73]. These *Random Forest Decision Trees* are prepared by combining the concept of bagging [73], and the random subspace [220]. It is mainly used in different applications [228, 451, 482].

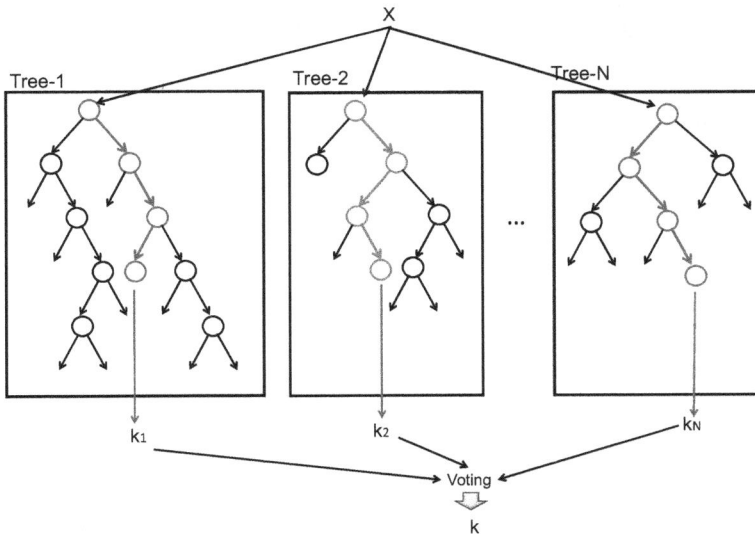

FIGURE 3.11: A *Random Forest* prepared by multiple *Decision Trees*.

Decision Tree and *Decision Forest* classifiers are also considered as *non-black-box* classifiers because of visible logic rules; this is the main essence of them as naïve readers can even understand why a particular instance is classified into a specific class. [137] used *Decision Forest* classifier called *Random Forest* and applied it on Intra-cranial *EEG* data set for selecting the intra-cranial channels to detect seizure early. The *Random Forest* provides 93.8% of accuracy. On the dataset of *ECoG* having 76 implanted electrodes, 64 are non-invasive, and 12 are invasive, and a *Decision Forest* named *Systematic Forest* has been used. This detected the seizure with 100% accuracy, [478].

3.3.1.4   Support vector machine

SVM was proposed by Vapnik [110]; it is a prominently used classifier for both regression and classification purposes [368]. It divides the data into two classes: C_1 and C_2 by selecting the hyperplane that linearly separates them. With this hyperplane, the *SVM* calculates the best coefficients that detach the classes. Its primary purpose is to explore the most suitable line that reduces the classification error for hidden records.

This has been widely used in disease detection and prediction, particularly in seizure detection. For example, *SVM* is used by [579] for patient-specific seizure detection with time-domain, frequency-domain, time-frequency, and non-linear features. *SVM* is used by [93] two popular data sets – *CHB-MIT* and *Bonn University* for detecting the seizure; they found an accuracy of 92.30% and 99.33%, respectively.

3.3.1.5   K-Nearest Neighbour

k-NN is a lazy, lightweight, but effective learning classification technique in *ML*, [13]. Typically, it is considered when all the attributes are numerical, but it can also apply to categorical attributes. For example, in a dataset, three records (rows), two of them are labeled, say *Yes* or *No*, but the third record is unlabelled [274, 446]. This case classifies the data based on the *Euclidean* distance [207] function and predicts the unlabelled (hidden) attribute by following two steps. Firstly, it searches for k training records nearest to the hidden records. Secondly, it picks the most frequently occurring classification for these instances. In seizure detection, this classifier has been used; for example, *k-NN* [184] proposed a method to predict the seizure and remove the computational complexity.

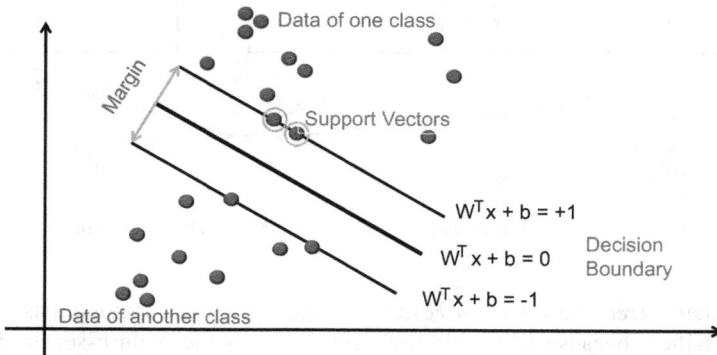

FIGURE 3.12: A training data set linearly separated by *SVM*.

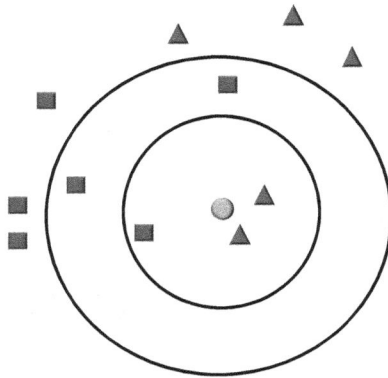

FIGURE 3.13: A k-Nearest Neighbour with different classes.

3.3.1.6   Artificial neural network

The human brain inspires the *ANN* concept as the human brain consists of 100 billion neurons, and these are interconnected to each other. Similarly, it processes the data in multiple hidden phases, and these phases are called neurons. In *ANN*, the network nodes are connected by links, and each link is associated with an associated weight, and they interact with each other in different layers. *ANN* comprises different layers, including an input layer, a hidden layer, and the output layer [207, 509]. The hidden phases are transient and have a probabilistic nature. *ANN* consists of inputs and their weights. Each hidden phase behaves as a bridge between the output of one layer and the input of another layer, and each process intends to learn from errors. The weighted inputs are then transformed into a single value using an activation function. Then the unique value is compared to the threshold(s) to determine the classification result [304, 552]. Like the human brain, input weights can be adjusted/learned in *ANN* to compensate classification errors. A general example of *ANN*, Figure 3.14 represents one input layer with n neurons, p hidden layers with n_1, n_2,...,np neurons in each layer, and one output layer with mn neurons. These numbers (n, n_1, n_2, n_p, mn) could be different.

3.3.2   Unsupervised learning methods

In *ML*, *ULM* indicate the patterns from the data sets that are neither classified nor labeled. The algorithms are used to organize them, based on their similarities and differences. It is more complicated than the *SLM*.

3.3.2.1   Clustering

Clustering is the most popular *ULM* method and is potentially applied for the pattern discovery process from the unstructured data set. It is applicable when the dataset does not have any target or class attribute, and no predefined grouping is found [569].

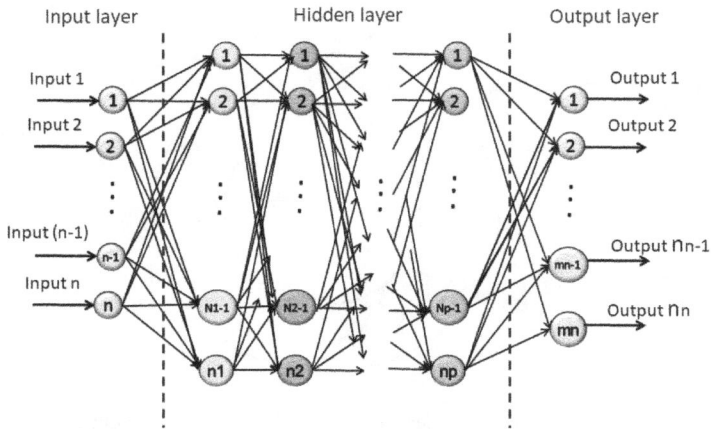

FIGURE 3.14: An *ANN* with multiple layers.

The data set is divided into clusters, and each cluster is a group of data objects based on similarities in some sense or characteristics in another [156]. A suitable *Clustering* method produces high-quality clusters to ensure that the inter-cluster similarity is low. The intra-cluster similarity is high; in other words, members of a cluster are more like each other than members of different clusters. Process clusters provide high-quality clusters to ensure that the inter-cluster similarity is less and higher in the intra-cluster. Alternatively, a cluster's objects are more similar to each other than similar to different clusters. *Clustering* has also been significantly applied to various applications [19]; it is also used on *EEG* data sets to detect seizures [61, 594, 469].

3.3.2.2   k-means

The *k-Means* algorithm is also one of the most popular *ULMs* for creating clusters. Considering k the number of groups that the user needs, done in n records in the data set D. The main idea is to define k centroids, one for each group. These centroids must be placed intelligently; the result depends on that; the best option is to put them as far apart as possible. The next step is to take each point that belongs to a given data set and associate it with the closest centroid. For each centroid, its position is recalculated from any distance function such as a Euclidean or a Cosine [22, 207].

The significant disadvantage of the k-means algorithm is that the user is limited to entering the desired number of clusters (e.g., $k = 10$). The final group does not represent a globally optimum result. Only the local and the last groups may arise from differences in the initial groups chosen randomly.

3.3.2.3   Genetic clustering

Genetic Clustering is a heuristic search that mimics the biological process. It is designed in five phases: initial population, fitness function, selection, crossing, and mutation. It starts with randomly generated states, and these states satisfy the problem.

The fitness function produces the next generation of states. A useful fitness function should return to a better condition. The fitness function scores each state. The probability of being chosen for breeding is based on the physical fitness score. In selection, two pairs are randomly selected for breeding. Selection is based on the fitness score. Each pair to be matched at a crossover point is chosen at random within the bit string. Exchanges between parents create offsprings at the crossing point. The population is diverse early in the process. This makes the crossover large initially; however, it settles into future generations. In mutation, each bit string location can be subject to mutation with a small random probability [330]. The basic principle is listed in 10 steps, Table 3.4.

TABLE 3.4: Genetic clustering algorithm.

Step	Instruction
1	t=0
2	Initialize p(t) population
3	Compute fitness p(t)
4	t=t+1
5	If the termination criterion achieved, go to *Step 10*
6	Select p(t) from p(t-1)
7	Crossover p(t)
8	Mutate p(t)
9	Go to *Step 3*
10	Output best and stop

3.4 Epileptic seizure detection

A brief overview of using *ML* for different epileptic seizure detection challenges has been done. Some revised examples of challenges are detection initiation, attack localization, imbalanced data set attack detection, among others.

3.4.1 Onset of seizure detection

ML methods are potentially applied at the beginning of seizure detection. They can provide an early alarm before the seizure occurs with automated detection; the doctor can be alerted when the seizure occurs. This detection method is very acceptable because, due to the lengthy *EEG* recordings, it is challenging to identify where the seizures started from and ended. Ultimately, seizure onset detection is also useful in determining brain locations that are effected by seizures. The medical team can easily monitor the activities during the seizure and the patient's responses. Since, *EEG* activities are of great help for neuro-experts to arrive at conclusions for further courses of action researchers [161, 257, 363, 444, 474, 196] have conducted several studies on this.

3.4.2   Quick seizure detection

Quick or fast seizure detection can be done by dividing the *EEG* dataset into shorter epochs based on time duration. This helps in creating future records in shorter durations of time called epochs. However, these epochs are non-overlapping datasets and in descending order which help to develop different datasets of different time frames, and these are further fed as inputs to the *ML* classifiers [479, 480]. At each epoch, the model's accuracy is tested once we get the maximum accuracy in a shorter epoch; the same has been used for seizure detection, and future records are created. This method is also significant for seizure prediction. For example, if a patient is experiencing an onset and under observation for 10 minutes, detecting the seizure will take the same duration. But after applying epoch reduction, if the seizure is detected in a minute, the future record is built in a minute's recording. Based on the training dataset, it will save time for future fast detection of seizures.

3.4.3   Seizure detection on class imbalance *EEG* dataset

A class imbalance is the most common problem in clinical datasets, a severe concern for data scientists while analyzing the dataset using available *ML* classifiers. The *EEG* recordings are of long duration, and during that, the seizure is for a few seconds. To recognize the actual seizure fluctuations in *EEG* signals is a complicated task. Traditionally, in the hospitals, *Epilepsy Monitoring Units (EMU)*, while detecting the seizure, made a mistake because they do onset seizure monitoring. As usual, the epileptic patient dataset is always imbalanced as seizure monitoring lasts for a long time, and in this period, the seizure duration occurrence is for a few seconds. Hence, there is a high probability of missing the neuro-technician's actual seizure timing, which made *ML* classifiers make mistakes due to bias. When bias occurs the classifier gets inclined towards the highly skewed data. As a result, it declares a seizure patient as a non-seizure one [477]. Several studies have been done to manage this issue in real-world scenarios, and it is found that an ensemble of classifiers approach is more effective than others, [178]. Researchers used different *ML* classifiers in the detection of epileptic seizures on an imbalanced dataset. [60] applied *ANN* along with weighted cost functions to the confusion matrix on an imbalanced *EEG* data set, and they obtained 86% detection rate. An imbalanced dataset, under-sampling with *SVM*, had been done achieving 97.3% accuracy [147]. *SMOTE* [92], a popular technique for imbalanced datasets, has been used with *RUSTBOST* [277] for detecting the seizure in an imbalanced dataset and obtained 97% accuracy.

3.4.4   Seizure localization

The brain is the most complex organ, constituting billions of nerves. The brain is divided into four major lobes [9, 394] – frontal, occipital, parietal, and temporal. The insula is the fifth lobe, deeply located between the temporal and parietal lobes. From the outer structure of the cerebral hemisphere, they are not separately apparent. The motive behind explaining these details is that seizure detection is not the only task in Epilepsy; identifying the correct position/location of the seizure(s) is also a critical challenge for the Neurologist's/Neurosurgeon's course of action. In this challenge, *ML* classifiers are quite helpful, particularly *non-black-box* classifiers such as *Decision Tree* and *Decision Forest*, because they provide the logic rules [480, 483] since the *EEG* electrodes/channels are implanted by the 10–20 *International System* [282].

[7] applied non-linear multi-way trucker kernels for seizure location [322] localize the seizures on the *EEG* dataset of 10s durations from *Karuniya University*. They have taken a small data set size because *EEG* recordings usually takes long time durations. If the data set taken is significant; then, the results are better. No one has claimed the exact percentage of the lobe damage by a seizure in these studies. However, results provided by [476, 480] showed that using *Decision Forest* approaches – *Systematic Forest* (*SysFor*) and *Forest CERN* with the help of sensible logic rules can help in identifying the percentage of seizure affected brain hemispheres.

3.4.5   Challenges in seizure detection

Typically, seizure monitoring is done by *EEG* and *ECoG* media. Just *ML* classifiers are not sufficient to detect the seizure. Therefore, some pre-requisites are needed, such as exploring the relevant and efficient statistical features from the raw *EEG/ECoG* signals. The data scientists always make sure that these features are neither more nor less; in both the scenarios, the dimensions of the data set suffer, which impacts the accuracy and computational cost. The literature reveals some have taken heaps of features above 65 in number, and some have taken just a single feature like line length and energy. In both cases, when a single feature is applied to all the electrodes, this multiplexer produces a high dataset dimension and this is a problem for the *ML* algorithms. Due to the long duration of *EEG* recordings, the number of records are in millions, and after multiplexing, the attribute size increases. If there are 76 electrode values and 65 used features, then the total attribute size is 76×65 = 4,940. This is a high dimensional dataset. There is a high chance of a misclassification error due to which some of the standard *ML* classifiers are not successful. Also, the computation cost of the classifier suffers heavily. On the contrary, if just one or two features are applied to the *EEG* dataset, then the produced dataset will have a low attribute size. This results, in poor knowledge discovery from the *EEG* signals and seizure information from the scalp. Hence, both extremes are dangerous. Considering a group of relevant features, could help manage the dimensionality of the dataset and the computational cost of the classifier. Although, the limitation, is that the number of features is not yet fixed.

Due to the advancement in technologies, several machine learning algorithms are designed; some are freely available as *ML* tools like *WEKA* [201], while some are commercial tools like *MATLAB*® *Toolbox* kit [218]. Therefore, for data scientists, it is a very decisive step to select the most appropriate classifier that could perform more effectively. From the analysis of different patient *EEG* datasets, it has been noted that the *non-black-box* classifier outperforms [479, 483]. They provide logic rules that help explore different patterns and majority voting methods, and their accuracy is also considerable.

3.5   Case study

An *EEG* recording is the most used method for monitoring brain activity. These recordings play a vital role in *ML* classifiers to explore novel methods for seizure detection in different ways, such as seizure onset detection, quick seizure detection, patient seizure detection, and seizure localization. The significance of publicly available datasets is that they provide a benchmark to analyze and compare other results. In the following section, the popular datasets that are widely used on Epilepsy will be described.

3.5.1   Child hospital *Boston-Massachusetts Institute of Technology* Dataset

This *Child Hospital Boston-Massachusetts Institute of Technology (CHB-MIT)* dataset is publicly available on the webserver of physionet. In the past few years it has been significantly used in seizure detection experiments particularly with machine learning algorithms. This dataset had been gathered from 24 patients' *EEG* recordings, comprising both *non-seizure* and *seizure* ones in European data format (.edf), representing the spikes with seizure onsets and ending moments.

Apart from the *CHB-MIT* dataset, others such as *Epilepsia, BONN, Freiburg,* and *Flint Hill* have also been prominently applied in the epileptic seizure detection process, as shown in Table 3.6.

The classification of seizure detection by different classifiers is carried out as discussed in Section 3.3. It requires four crucial components:

Class attribute *(CA)* is a target attribute, which is discrete in nature and represents distinct values, termed as class-values (CA_i). Typically, in the epilepsy dataset, the class values are described as *seizure* or *non seizure*.

Non-Class attributes are independent predictors for a data set, e.g., the data sets contain n *non-class attributes* and each feature presents different statistical information of brain signals.

Training data set contains both *non-class attributes* and *class attributes*, whose values are not hidden. The *ML* classifier is applied to it.

Testing data set is used to detect the performance of a classifier. This is done by using n-fold *Cross-Validation (CV)* (mostly ten fold). In 10 fold validation, CV data is trained and validated for 10 times.

The performance of the classifiers is evaluated and computed by using the *Confusion Matrix* - based evaluation matrix parameters such as precision, recall, and

TABLE 3.5: *CHB-MIT* epilepsy dataset summary.

S. No.	ID	Age	Sex	No. Channels	No. Seizure	Seizure Duration (mm:ss)
1	chb01	11	F	23	7	7:12
2	chb02	11	M	23	3	2:50
3	chb03	14	F	23	7	5:40
4	chb04	22	F	23	4	4:00
5	chb05	07	F	23	5	9:00
6	chb06	1.5	F	23	10	2:00
7	chb07	14.5	F	23	3	5:10
8	chb08	3.5	F	23	5	15:10
9	chb09	10	F	21	4	4:00
10	chb10	03	F	23	7	6:50
11	chb11	12	F	23	3	13:20
12	chb12	02	F	23	27	14:50
13	chb13	03	F	18	12	8:10
14	chb14	09	F	23	8	2:30
15	chb17	12	F	23	3	4:40
12	chb18	18	F	23	6	4:50
13	chb19	19	F	23	3	3:40
14	chb20	06	F	23	8	3:30
15	chb21	13	F	23	4	3:10
16	chb22	09	F	23	3	3:10
17	chb23	06	F	23	7	6:40

TABLE 3.6: Datasets.

Dataset	Year	Num of subjects	Num of hours	Num of Seizure	Num of Electrodes	EEG type	Sampling rate (Hz)
Epilepsiae [227]	2014	275	300,000	2,662	125	sEEG iEEG	250– 2500
CHB-MIT [474]	2009	23	1,000	198	23–26	sEEG	256
Freiburg [561]	2003	21	582	87	128	iEEG	256
Flint Hill [380]	2001	10	1,419	49	48–64	iEEG	240
BONN [26]	2001	5	35	5	2	sEEG iEEG	173.61

F-measure [410, 479, 481]. It is based on four possible classification outcomes, Table 3.7.

Precision is the ratio of true positives to the cases that are predicted as positive. It is the percentage of selected cases that are correct. *Recall* is the ratio of true positives to the cases that are positive. It is the percentage of correct cases that are selected.

TABLE 3.7: Possible classification outcomes.

Acronym	Definition	Description
TP	True Positive	Positive and predicted positive
TN	True Negative	Negative and predicted negative
FN	False Negative	Positive but predicted to be negative
FP	False Positive	Negative but predicted to be positive

TABLE 3.8: Suitable classifier for seizure detection.

Patient ID	Data Set	Classifier	Accuracy	Precision	Recall	F-measure
P1	$D_1 - 10s$	Decision Tree	99.1	83.33	64.1	72.46
		SVM	99.4	90.63	74.36	81.69
		kNN	99.4	90.63	74.36	81.69
		Ensemble	99.5	96.67	74.36	**84.06**
	$D_2 - 0.5s$	Decision Tree	99.1	81.26	67.15	73.53
		SVM	99.4	93.18	74.12	82.56
		kNN	99.3	95.45	67.37	78.99
		Ensemble	99.4	91.13	78.43	**84.3**
P2	$D_3 - 10s$	Decision Tree	98.9	71.88	60.53	65.71
		SVM	98.8	65.79	65.79	65.79
		kNN	98.7	64.71	57.89	61.11
		Ensemble	99.2	88.89	63.16	**73.85**
	$D_4 - 0.5s$	Decision Tree	99.1	77.82	70.24	73.84
		SVM	99.4	93.21	74.45	82.78
		K-NN	99.3	96.18	66.92	78.93
		Ensemble	99.4	90.93	77.65	**83.77**

From Table 3.8 and Figure 3.15, an analysis of results for all four data sets of both the patients revealed that *SVM* is dominates *kNN*. In three data sets, the accuracy and *F*-measure values of *SVM* are higher compared to *kNN*. *kNN* does not perform well in terms of accuracy and the *F*-measure because it has too many data points. A high dimension data set of 208 attributes and 50,400 records was used. The *black-box* classifiers are not capable of interpreting classification steps performed at several class values. As a result, they have very limited meaningful patterns forming them; it is difficult to conclude discovery of knowledge. On the contrary, a *non-black-box* classifier can acquire knowledge and expose it in a human-understandable format. Two *non-black-box* classifiers: *Decision Tree* and *Decision Forrest* were compared. Our experimental results show that the *F*-measure of the *Decision Forest* classifier is much better than that of a single *Decision Tree* (see Table 3.8 and Figure 3.15).

From the result of both patient data sets shown in Table 3.8, the *F-measure* value of the *ensemble* classifier outperforms the decision tree, as shown in Figure 3.15.

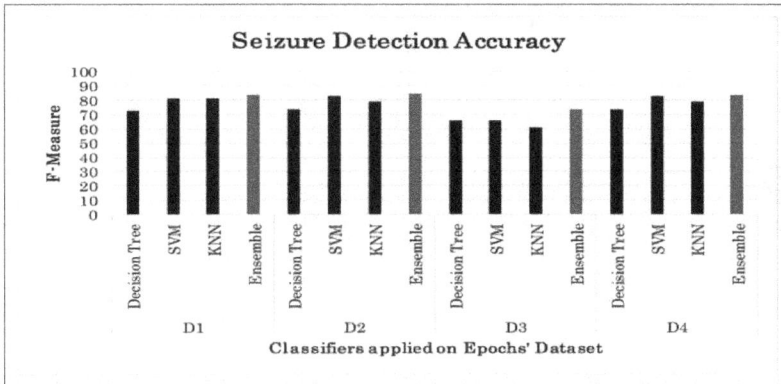

FIGURE 3.15: Classifiers comparison for seizure detection.

In 10 secs the epoch length data set of the patient (P_1), the *F-measure* value of the *Decision Forest* classifier is 84.06, followed by a *Decision Tree* value of 72.46, which is lower in comparison to the ensemble value because it generates a limited number of logic rules with a lower accuracy rate. *Decision forest* generates a set of logic rules; each tree of a *decision forest* behaves as a classifier due to this reason; it provides more logic rules. As a result, we get high performance in terms of classification accuracy with a high *F-measure*.

Since one of its classifiers is an ensemble, it generates a set of logic rules. As a result, it is widely used for knowledge discovery purposes. *SVM* vs *kNN*. From Table 3.8 and Figure 3.15, we analyze the results for all four data sets of both the patients and find that *SVM* dominates *kNN*. In three data sets, the accuracy and F-measure values of *SVM* are higher compared to *K-NN* values. Here, *kNN* does not perform well in terms of accuracy and F-measures because the data set has too many data cells. We have used a high dimension data set of 208 attributes and 50,400 records. However, in a single data set, each accuracy value is 99.1 and F-measure is 81.69, respectively.

3.6 Conclusions

ML applications are not limited. They are significantly and powerfully used in different real-world scenarios. ML is an actively adopted method by a *medical science* team with the *data scientist* to diagnose and intervene. Similarly, in Epilepsy, it has been an applied technology as the collected *EEG* dataset is versatile, complex, time-dependent, non-stationary, and chaotic. With these tedious characteristics, simple signal processing methods are insufficient to extract meaningful information. *ML* techniques show promising results in seizure onset detection, fast detection, early detection, seizure localization, and more. *ML* techniques have not been significantly used to discover the group of anti-epileptic drugs for a patient. They depend on factors including demographics, age, gender, hormones, genetic history, reaction to a particular drug and more [520].

Indeed, every time all the classifiers don't behave well for all types of data sets. The performance of a classifier also depends on the data set dimensions. Overall, it is estimated that the *ensemble* classifier works better than the *black-box* classifiers in terms of accuracy and knowledge discovery. Generally, a *non-black-box* classifier (ensemble) outperforms other *black-box* classifiers to the best of our knowledge. Even the *ensemble* performs better than a single *decision tree*, which is a *non-black-box* classifier.

False detection is one of the main concerns in the existing *ML* classifiers that start giving alarms for more than one seizure type, and are probably the major impediment for clinical application. Most classifiers were applied and tested on the available dataset due to heaps of records. The false detections were due to reasons like high skewness towards one class. In the Epilepsy Monitoring Unit, most patient recordings were less inclined towards actual seizure, so again, it is likely that false positives were even higher. Despite these limitations, these techniques have been implemented with a ubiquitous system in the hospital for onset of patient-specific seizure detection.

4

Simultaneous Evaluation of Children Epileptic Encephalopathies with Long-Term EEG via Space-Time Dynamic Entropies

Ricardo Zavala-Yoé* and *Ricardo A Ramirez-Mendoza*

4.1 Introduction

Epileptic seizures are expressions of epilepsy. Seizures are violent discharges of electrical activity in the brain that temporarily affect how it works. Here, violence means sudden interruption in the normal functioning of the brain. They can manifest as a "smooth" loss of consciousness (as in absences seizures) or, conversely, in the case of falls.

There are four identified seizure phases: (a) Pre-ictal, which refers to the state immediately before the actual discharge; (b) Ictal, relates to the state when the actual seizure happens; (c) Postictal refers to the stage shortly after the discharging event; (d) Interictal, means the lapse between seizures [361], [456], [332], [167], [454]. In this work, we only consider the first three of them.

The International League Against Epilepsy (ILAE) defines Epilepsy as a disorder of the brain characterized by an enduring predisposition to generate epileptic seizures, and by the neurobiological, cognitive, psychological, and social consequences of this condition [56], [332], [456], [167], [454]. The latter require the occurrence of at least one epileptic seizure. In addition, a syndrome describes a disorder in which a certain combination of characteristics regularly occur. ILAE defines epileptic encephalopathy (EE) as the state where the epileptic event itself is a factor for cognitive and behavioral impairments seen in severe epilepsy, beyond that expected from underlying pathology alone [456], [542], [501], [135], [167], [454]. In this spirit, ILAE coined the term *drug resistant* to designate the reluctance of the affection to be treated with standard AED. Typical examples of EE are Doose and Lennox-Gastaut syndromes (DS and LGS, respectively). They usually are drug resistant and recommending definitive treatments becomes hard and compromising. From these definitions of terms, it can be inferred that we deal with complex affections (reflected also as complex mathematical entities). So, a quantitative analysis of these

School of Engineering and Sciences, Tecnologico de Monterrey, Monterrey, Mexico.
* Corresponding author: rzavalay@tec.mx

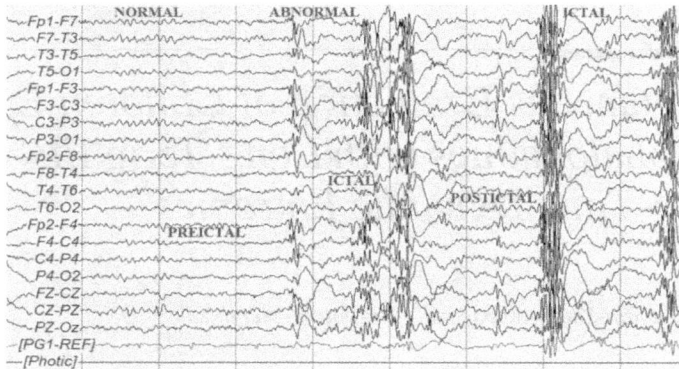

FIGURE 4.1: Stages of a seizure: Preictal (state prior to a seizure), ictal (development of the seizure), postictal (recuperation).

EE by means of their corresponding EEGs has to be considered as very relevant. Although some quantitative techniques have been applied to various brain diseases, there is still a lack of math attention to EE (and more to DS and LGS, excluding our contributions). That is why we offer to use a collection of our parameters and graphs to support an objective analysis of EEG in the case of DS and LGS.

4.1.1 The Doose syndrome

Since the 60's, Hermann Doose, German neuropediatrician, investigated the characteristics of a previously incompletely understood child epilepsy syndrome epitomized by a wide heterogeneity of seizures. The most frequent are jerks, jerks followed by falls, drop attacks, absences with the possibility of generalized tonic-clonic seizures too. Something frustrating is the fact that at the beginning of the patient's life, the health and behavior may be normal, but as time goes by, the evolution of this illness reflects peculiar patterns in the EEG. Typically found patterns are generalized spike and polyspike waves, and 4–7 rhythms/s with bursts [456], [361], [135]. It has been registered that 1%–2% of all children with epilepsy constitute DS. This rare disorder onsets classically from 7 months to 6 years [255], [456], [361], [135], [501], [542].

4.1.2 The Lennox-Gastaut syndrome

This syndrome can originate due to many causes, nevertheless about 33%–50% of all cases may be associated to some related sickness or even to brain damage. This syndrome affects about 3% of all children that suffer from epilepsy although about 33% of the patients that deal with this disease do not show any symptom at the beginning. This condition is often confused with DS because LGS is also characterized by many types of seizures that can be very aggressive. Onset is between 2 and 8 years of age, peculiarly with drop head and atonic seizures It is well known that myoclonic, focal, tonic-clonic, tonic, astatic seizures as well as atypical absences can also show up together in a patient. The EEG findings unfold focal and multifocal sharp slow waves with a pronounced tendency to spread out. However, the main focus of all discharges is the frontal lobe with a rapid spread to the lateral lobes. LGS is distinguished by three features:

- The main EEG findings are slow spikes.

- A wide multiplicity of seizures takes place during sleep.

- Intellectual disability.

The definitions and elucidations given above permit the expectation that DS and LGS are drug resistant (DR) and multifocal affections. These facts imply that a profusion of AED must be tested and many EEG studies have to be collected [456], [361], [501], [542], [135], [167], [454], [56], [62].

4.1.3 Raison d'être

Two perspectives can be identified in modelling and analysis of EEG: (a) Deterministic non-linear dynamical systems (Chaos-based theory) and (b) Stochastic models [180], [221], [505], [261], [510], [577]. Since every condition is patient-dependent, it is very difficult (if not impossible) to find a single model that can mathematically characterize a given disease for all possible cases. There have been some reports about math models for some common or unspecified types of epilepsies. The results are conservative and particular, but a generalized analytical structure is still missing. It has been shown (as it could be expected) that normal (non-epileptic) EEG-data tends to exhibit a normal distribution with a linear behavior (in the sense of a quartile-quartile plot [51]. In contrast, abnormal EEG, as in the case of epilepsy, tends to show non-normal distributions with a non-linear structure (in the sense of a quartile-quartile plot) [586], [585], [261], [587]. Exploring particular non-linear dynamical models results is then very restrictive because such a model (if any) works for a specific patient for a certain time lapse because—obviously—we would need to involve the time-varying nature of data in such dynamical models. Then, dealing with mathematical structures that are constrained is not reliable up until now. We have proposed a way to circumvent the above mentioned restrictions using nonlinear statistics referred to as time series entropies or time series complexity measures [398], [101], [433], [340]. This stochastic perspective for any time series does not have any problem as explained before. As known, a time series is a realization of a stochastic process and each EEG channel is represented by a time series, so several databases of children with epilepsy were investigated in [584]-[583]. The characteristics studied were normality (in distributional sense), stationarity and linearity. Our results also revealed that healthy EEG data tends to be normally distributed as well as being linear and stationary, in line with some other works ([586] and references therein). Conversely, our EEG-data was stationary, normal (in distributional sense), and nonlinear (with respect to a quantile-quantile plot). Statistical testing of linearity and stationarity versus nonlinearity and non-stationarity is not a minor task [340], [586], [584] and nonlinearity could not be proven in the sense of classical works. Ergo, determining a well grounded and extensive stochastic model is not feasible for DS and LGS. In view of this, we propose to work with a "combined" strategy, i.e., we proposed to use nonlinear statistics, also known as complexity measures [584]-[583]. Our set of complexity measures is based on seminal works found in [398], [433], [101], [497], [111], [566]. It was already mentioned that DS and LGS are drug resistant diseases and this implies that the number of EEGs practiced on a child may be high. If, for instance, seizures onset in a child at the age of 2, when the child becomes 11 years old, there will be 9 EEG records in the case of a yearly prescription. At this point our investigation questions (posed now in a single query) arise: How to analyze all the information contained in all the EEG records in a handy way? We must contemplate that, in order to Figure out the health state of the child, the neurologist could review just a few of the EEG records collected by the parents. But also, this physician may want to study the last EEG performed on the child; or it may be just the first. Also, he/she could deny taking into account all EEG data stored for years, ordering a new one. All this worsens if more than one neurologist is needed over time, which would not be strange in EE like DS and LGS. An objective procedure to deal with our research questions is necessary, on behalf of children, parents and clinicians.

4.2 Methods: subjects and metrics for DS and LGS

This section describes the research method, the subjects and the employed metrics.

4.2.1 Conditions

This section encompasses several works [29–34] to show how mathematics can help to answer investigative questions. Bearing in mind that the patients taken into account here suffer a type of an EE (i.e., DS or LGS), supplementary considerations (SC) are shown next [312], [334], [349], [336], [559], [555], [554]:

- Patients are infants with an early onset of seizures.

- Patients have a long story of suffering a drug resistant condition (i.e., about 10 years).

- Seizures manifest as multifocal discharges.

- Subjects have responded to medical therapies.

- Intending to track appropriate medical care without interruption, patients had to be treated preponderantly in only one hospital.

These constraints limit the number of potential candidates for the study even more. Accordingly, we design a pilot study developed in [584]-[583] that helps neurologists to contend with grave EE cases. It is common knowledge that a pilot study depicts an essential stage of the exploration process with the aim of assessing the viability of applying a small-scale study to a larger one. A pilot study does not provide any statistical justification for the time being [294] but at this point, we reflect that our patients represent serious cases of a very aggressive disorder that also manifests in a very complex dynamic as a mathematical entity. As far as we are concerned, there are no excluded contributions in this field [584]-[583]. It must also be noted that a further labyrinth to the SC given above, is the fact that in developing countries complying with medical treatments in public children hospitals may be very byzantine [17, 19, 21]. As can be realized, obtaining a larger number of patients satisfying all these requirements is quite arduous. So, our pilot study is composed of a case series of five subjects. Four suffer a case of EE with the abovementioned complications (SC); all of them are referred to as **drug resistant epileptic encephalopathies (DREES)** [586]. We also have a normal (non-epileptic) patient for comparison purposes.

4.2.2 Subjects

The study group of subjects is made up of five children: four are affected by LGS or DS or even a combination of them. The fifth is normal (non-epileptic affection) and its EEG recordings were used as a reference. Infants A and B were born in 2002; children C, D, and E in 2001, 2003, and 2006, respectively. In line with the guidelines of the Declaration of Helsinki, our ex post facto research does not raise any ethical concerns beside appropriate anonymization. Consequently, every personal detail was kept anonymous, and only numerical raw data and medications were handled.

4.2.3 Antiepileptic drugs (AED) prescribed to the subjects

The AED consumed by the patients are shown in Table 4.1. This Table is taken from [585] and [586]. Other information as side/adverse effects, dosages, pharmacological interactions can be reviewed in [136], [361], [559], [56], [336], [555], [554].

TABLE 4.1: Abbreviation for the AED consumed by patients A-D.

AED	Abbrev.	AED	Abbrev.
Imipramine	IMI	Ethosuximide	ESM
Piracetam	PA	Prednisone	PSE
Magnesium valproate	VPA+	Atomoxetine	ATX
Topiramate	TPM	Midazolam	MDZ
Clobazam	CLB	Clonazepam	CZP
Valproate sodium	VPA	Zonisamide	ZNS
Lamotrigina	LTG	Clorasepate dipotassium	CZP
Levetiracetam	LEV	Phenobarbital	PB
Lacosamide	LCM	Primidone	PRM

4.2.4 Patient A

The first child (called A) was initially diagnosed as DS but as time went, the pathology seemed to be transformed to LGS with several disagreements by neurologists. The last diagnosis was DS as a result of the EEG findings. The principal seizures source is located in the frontal lobe with a rapid dispersion to all brain sections. This child was born in 2002. The DREE onsets at 4 years old as absence seizures. At the age of 5 (in 2007), shivers were very characteristic but this condition worsened as heads dropped when it was necessary to use a helmet [585], [586], [583], [588], [361]. In 2007, six AED were already in use but with poor success (see Table 4.2). Due to this, fourteen more AED were included in the group [136], [361], [336]. In spite of this, seizures did not improve, neither in intensity nor in number. Moreover, although the child had already suffered myoclonic, dropping heads and absence seizures, new types of them showed up (drops, night eyelid myoclonia, and more). The most critical period for this child was in 2014 when even 80 convulsions a day were displayed. Actually, the number of attacks reached 80 a day. So, it was mandatory to take the child to a hospital emergency room. However, in spite of a clear deterioration, she could not be admitted due to administrative procedures. A palliative solution was to increase some AED dosage. After three months of fighting against seizures, the child was finally admitted and some adjustments were made in the AED. However, four months later, seizures worsened again and as a result of all these useless actions, the parents took their daughter to another hospital where IVIG (intravenous immune globulin) was supplied in 2015. This substance caused a very positive effect on the child's health and a very clear improvement in her life was evident. Around the same time IVIG was provided, although cannabidiol (CBD) [331], [225] was also suggested as a future alternative treatment [586]. The reason for this was that CBD has demonstrated success in very severe cases of DREES. Accessible EEG were recorded in 2008, 2010, 2011 and 2013; absent years were not included in this investigation for administrative problems as reported in [585], [586]. In Tables 4.2, and 4.3, $\sqrt{}$ means relative good control of seizures and × means poor/no control. ∗ indicates the year in which an EEG study was recorded.

TABLE 4.2: Anticonvulsants per year for patient A.

Anticonvulsant	Year/period	Seizures
IMI,PM	2006	×
VPA+,TPM,CLB,VPA	2007	×
VPA,LTG,TPM,VPA+,CLB,LEV,ATX,ESM,PSE,MDZ	2008*	√
TPM,LEV,LTG,PSE,ESM,CZP,ZNS,	2009	×
ZNS,ESM,CZP,LEV,CZP	2010*	×
CZP,LEV,LTG,ESM,PB	2011*	×
LCM,ESM,LEV,LTG,CZP	2012	×
LCM,LEV,LTG,PRM,CZP,Q10,ESM	2013a*	√
LEV,ESM,LCM,LTG,CZP	2013b*	√
LEV,ESM,LTG,CLB, *IVIG*	2014	√
LEV,ESM,LTG,CLB, *IVIG*	2015	√

TABLE 4.3: Anticonvulsants per period for patient B.

Anticonvulsant	Year	Comments	Seizures
VPA	2006a*	Onset of seizures, VPA prescribed	×
VPA	2006b*	Seizures improve a bit, VPA	√
VPA	2009*	Seizures continue, VPA	×
VPA	2011	None (VPA retired), seizures improve	√
VPA, LEV	2013*	LEV prescribed	√

4.2.5 Patient B

Child B was born in 2002 and he/she was identified as LGS from his/her early childhood. Seizures onset with frontal-temporal supply. EEG-database findings are featured by very intense multifocal, high voltage peak waves. Ictal activity manifests as mostly frontal and temporal. The AED consumed are shown in Table 4.1. Observe the contrast in AED between patient A and B. The EEGs accessible were recorded in July/August, 2006, 2009, and 2011, [513], [555], [554], [584]–[586].

4.2.6 Patient C

It was possible to retrieve three records from this child. They were recorded in 2005, 2006, 2007 and 2009. LEV, LTG, LTG and VPA were the principal AED. This subject was born in 2001. It seems that seizures start at the frontal lobe, [584]–[586], [56], [501], [255].

4.2.7 Patient D

He/she was born in 2003, and diagnosed with DS although some features of LGS manifested at seizure onset. The Seizure source was located in the frontal lobe. EEG database was collected from 2006 to 2014, although accessible records were made in 2006, 2010, and 2013. The main AED consumed were VPA, ESM, LEV and CZP. The focus of the seizures was not identified but was the frontal lobe in all likelihood [584]–[586], [555], [554].

4.2.8 Patient E

He/she was born in 2006 with no seizures problems. The EEG were used just for comparison purposes. The EEG databases were recorded while the child sat playing a computer game, [584]–[586].

4.2.9 EEG general information

All EEG data was acquired from different children hospitals. All of it was recorded from scalp in 32 channels-Grass Technologies Clinical Systems (Natus Technology 2015) according to the well known international 10–20 system; 7 mm, 50 μv calibration [456], [332], [426]. The following were the standard EEG channels used in hospitals for all patients: Fp1, Fp2, F3, F4, F7, F8, Fz, C4, C5, Cz, T3, T4, T5, T6, P3, P4, Pz, O1, O2 (Oz not included) at a sample frequency of 200 Hz, i.e., 5 ms. For all subjects with epilepsy all EEGs were sleep-deprived. Child E was awake while he/she was playing a video game on a computer. The same type of EEG acquisition device used for patients was also used in subject E. It should be mentioned that fast accidental events do not alter our calculations or graphs. Non-epileptic muscular occurrences last just for an instant and so chills, eye blinks, and others. do not affect calculations. In spite of having obtained good numerical results in all our studies, inspection of an experienced neurophysiologist is always wanted. Our conclusions were in line with expert positions.

4.2.10   Entropy metrics

Claude Shannon, mathematician and electrical engineer, also known as the "father of information theory" (1948), defined entropy of a time series as a measure of regularity; he coined this term to determine how repetitive or nearly repetitive a sampled signal is [466], [101], [398], [433]. In this sense, a sine wave and a square wave will have a very low complexity value (low entropy) while a random signal will have a high complexity (high entropy). A signal will be complex if its entropy is bigger than one, and regular or non-complex if such a value is less than one [585], [587], [586], [101], [398], [433]. Along the same lines, Pincus (1991) established the theory to appraise a measurement of uniformity or consistency [398], [433]. He was drawn to the idea of implementing that to clinical numerical records. The consequent statistic was named approximate entropy (ApEn). This statistic has been progressing and it has received different names hinging upon the advancement: sample entropy, SaEn [101], [398], [433], multiscale entropy, MSE [111], [566], our version of MSE [585], the so called composite multiscale entropy and our proposed bivariate MSE (BMSE) [585]-[583] as well as some others [298]. Thus, all these parameters have been designed to estimate the entropy (or complexity) of a sampled signal (as the EEG). High values of entropy (values bigger than 1) indicate that a signal is complex (a normal EEG, a random function is not regular nor periodic). Low numbers (smaller than 1) mean low complexity (high regularity as a sine wave). The above mentioned metrics (ApEn, SaEn, MSE, CMSE and MMME) were investigated in [101], [111], [566], [584]-[583]. There, it was shown that our version of the MSE was the most convenient to deal with a case of child epilepsy. Later, in the same works a case series was studied and in [584]-[583] a pilot study was described. Additionally in [584]-[583], a collection of dynamic complexity plots was studied offering graphical criteria and interpretations. It is notable to mention that all these algorithms and programs are self-produced with MATLAB® [517].

4.2.11   Modified MSE basic algorithm

This MSE algorithm presented by us in [585] is an amended version of the basic MSE calculation [111]. In the following example, a piece of a signal (i.e., a section of an EEG) will be analyzed. Assume that we take four samples of a certain channel of an EEG record. These samples are given as $X = [X(1), X(2), X(3), ..., X(L)]$ (micro volts) where L is the length of the time series which represent it. Now, define a subsample-rates vector as $\tau = [1, 2, ..., \tau_{max}]$. Notice that for $\tau = 1$ we have the original time series X. Let us define a new length m for vector u. Let us fix $m = 2$ with the purpose of storing m pieces of X in u as: $u(1) = [X(1), X(2)]$ and $u(2) = [X(3), X(4)]$. Now we have to find out how similar they are to each other. Obviously, as smaller is the distance between them, the more comparable they are (and the signal would tend to be regular). Thus, distances are $d(1) = |X(1) - X(3)|$ and $d(2) = |X(2) - X(4)|$. Now select the biggest difference for each pair of pieces, $max(d1, d2)$, $max(d3, d4)$, ... If $d(1) < r$ where r is a threshold, and we count this event as valid and a counter, say c is increased, i.e., $c = c + 1$. We proceed analogously for $d(2)$, and so on until finishing with all entries. Divide the latter by $(L - m + 1)$ and name this ratio c. Determine a logarithmic probability taking the natural logarithm of the aforementioned term for every c, adding them together at the end. Name this result Φ_m. Now compute a new logarithmic probability as before for sub vectors of length $m + 1$ and call it Φ_{m+1}. Finally, the complexity of this piece of the sampled signal will be given by the difference of the latter logarithmic probabilities, $\Phi_m - \Phi_{m+1}$. The latter complexity or entropy parameter is known as multiscale entropy (MSE). Since the latter was done for $\tau(1) = 1$, all the above presented tasks will be replicated for all the remaining values of the subsample rate vector $\tau = [1, 2, ..., \tau_{max}]$. At the end of the procedure, a collection of MSE values is plotted for each τ. This chart is referred to as the MSE complexity graph. Details about this algorithm can be seen in [585], [587], [586].

Below, a collection of MSE complexity plots are illustrated for a preictal, ictal and post ictal stage of a seizure.

In Figure 4.2 it can be appreciated that the algorithm just described was used to determine the complexity of a section of a certain EEG. This part of the EEG consists of a preictal, ictal and a postictal phase and are given (from top to bottom) in the left column of the image. In the second column, the MSE complexity plot shows that a relatively high complexity behavior is displayed in the first and third sections of this second column. This happens because first, the patient is about to suffer the seizure (preictal stage), then the seizure starts (ictal stage), and finally, the patient recovers (post ictal part). Notice how almost all values of the seizure complexity plot are less than 1, on the contrary with respect to the other two graphs.

4.2.12   Modified MSE algorithm

Below a procedure is illustrated for an EEG channel represented by a time series (vector X). The length of this series is L and is determined by the number of samples in the channel. A subsample vector is constructed starting with $\tau = 1$ up to τ_{max} using a step size of Δx. In this way, the algorithm is applied to each sub sampled vector at a rate fixed by vector τ. An additional variable m is used to examine X by means of length-m sub vectors u. X is a sub partition to construct vectors Y and from these, vectors u are constructed to compute similarities between pairs of sub

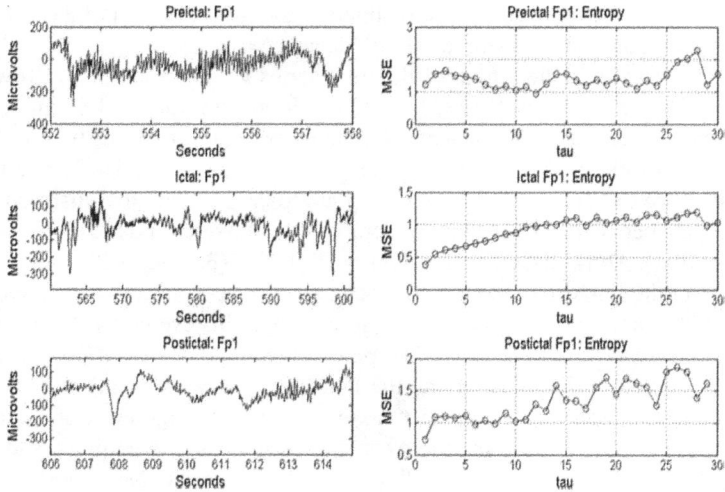

FIGURE 4.2: Channel Fp1 (frontal lobe). Seizure stages and their corresponding entropy plots.

vectors using a measure of distance d. The number of distances that are smaller than a threshold r are counted and added together for every piece u. The latter is repeated for next adjacent vectors u and a natural logarithmic probability is computed for each u (the original one and the adjacent one). The latter result defines the MSE for a given sample rate, τ. Notice that when $\tau(1) = 1$, the procedure is applied to the original time series (complete length L). This recurrent task is repeated for all vectors τ and thus a collection of MSE values is computed to build a MSE complexity plot (τ, MSE) [584]–[583].

Note: In Algorithm 1, # denotes "number of times".

4.2.13 MSE index

In Section 4.2.11, it was mentioned that a logarithmic probability is computed. This part consists of taking a natural logarithm of a ratio. If that ratio is formed by two identical numbers (up to decimal extent), then the natural logarithm of this will be ln(1)=0 and the complexity is null (see Algorithm 1). Thus, entropy values smaller than 1 mean low complexity and entropy values bigger than one mean high complexity. See Figure 4.2. As expected, this will not be the case for an aperiodic signal.

Example 1. The conception of implementing Algorithm 1 to epileptic encephalopathies as Doose and Lennox-Gastaut syndromes was presented in [585], [584]. There, subject A was investigated and it was possible to compare – by complexity plots – all records per brain zone at the same time. In this way, the worst year and the worst zone were immediately identified and these results were linked to the AED consumed (see illustration 4.3). Thus, a complete comparative study was presented in [29–35] in line with clinical interpretations.

Algorithm 1 MSE index (modified MSE)

Input: $X = [X(1), X(2), \ldots, X(L)]$, τ_{max}, $\Delta\tau$, m.

Output: Mean value of MSE per τ entry and a complexity plot (τ, MSE).

L $\leftarrow length(X)$

for $\tau = 1$ to τ_{max} step size $\Delta\tau$,
j=1 to L/τ, i=(j-1) to j*τ **do**

$Y(\tau) \leftarrow (1/\tau) \sum_i^j X(i)$
$r(Y(\tau)) \leftarrow 0.2\sigma(Y(\tau))$

    for p=1 to 2 **do**

        for q=1 to L-m+1 **do**

            $u(q) = \leftarrow [Y(q), Y(q+1), \ldots Y(q+m+1)]$

            $d(u(q), u(q+1) \leftarrow max_q = |u(q) - u(q+1)|$

            N $\leftarrow$ #(d¡r)

            $C(q) \leftarrow$ k/(L-m+1)

end for j
end for i

$\Phi(p) \leftarrow 1/(L-m+1) \sum_{q=1}^{L-m+1} C(q)$
m $\leftarrow$ m+1

        end for p

        $S(q) \leftarrow (\Phi(p) - \Phi(p+1)) = 1/(L-m+1) \sum_{q=1}^{L-m+1} \ln\left(\frac{C(q)}{C(q+1)}\right)$

        end for q

end for τ

MSE(q) $\leftarrow$ mean(S(q))
Plot(τ,MSE)

Example 2. Patient B data were examined as follows. The 23 channels of a 50-minutes EEG were divided into 5 time-sections, each of 10 minutes duration. It was possible to analyze the complete record for this brain portion in this way. Of course, all parameters are adjustable. As can be seen in image 4.4, a lot of information can be covered with the help of MSE indices. In this image it can be perceived that the lowest complexity values correspond to the curve that represents the first period (0–10s). The average MSE is approximately 0.2, indicating that this is a period with preponderant seizure brain activity. Bottom to top, the second regular curve is the one which depicts the period from 20s–30s. Following this way, the sequence is (40s–50s), (10s–20s) and (30s–40s). For this reason, the worst period encompasses

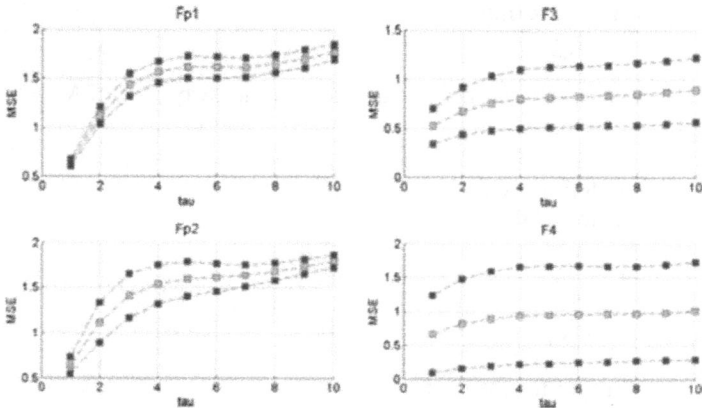

FIGURE 4.3: MSE indices plots that detect F4 as the most affected area (observe high data dispersion in the standard deviation curves above/below the MSE mean curve). The EEG portion lasts 5 minutes. This duration is adjustable and this computation also permits identifying the worst period.

the first ten seconds, and the best one runs from ten to twenty seconds. See the upward trend of all curves which means that despite the presence of continuous seizures, the child's organs struggle to behave as normally as possible.

In Figure 4.5, the mean of each MSE curve (picture 4.4) has been portrayed for each studied period: p0 = 0s–10s, p1 = 10s–20s, p2 = 20s–30s, p3 = 30s–40s and p4 = 40s–50s. Hence, what we explained about Figure 4.4 is true but we can consider that Figure 4.5 is a more condensed equivalent. The mean of all the MSE indices per period in that Figure is $\overline{MSE} = 0.76788$, quite below 1 and its standard deviation is $\sigma_{MSE} = 0.35525$.

Finally, in the case of MSE indices that provide information for the whole brain, it is very useful to produce their graph that shows the complexity of each brain region (see illustration 4.6). In such a diagram, the section of the brain (EEG channel) with the lowest/highest entropy value can be easily recognized.

4.2.14   BMSE and BMSE index: three dimensional complexity information

It has been shown that MSE indices produce a useful Figure for a determined lapse of time. Nevertheless, if this period is too long (half an hour, one hour or longer) computing and plotting MSE curves for all channels for several periods may take a long time (5–10 minutes, depending on data length as well).

A way to circumvent this problem is to create a set of MSE curves placed all together for a period of time; this means that a "slice" of MSE will show information for time period 1, next to it, a second MSE slice will provide information for the next time period and so on until the partition is finished for the entire time the EEG was

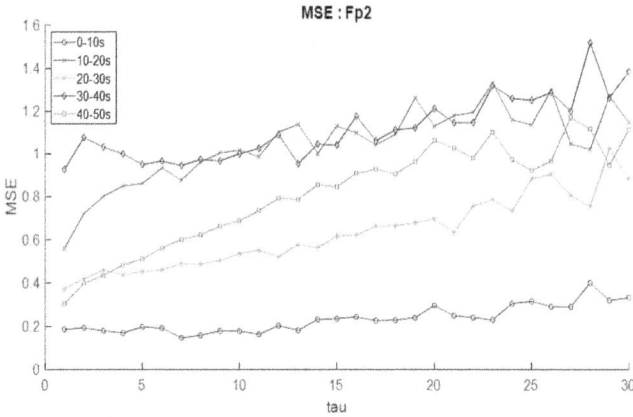

FIGURE 4.4: MSE indices per time period partition for channel Fp2 (patient B). The complete record lasts 52 seconds with 23 channels.

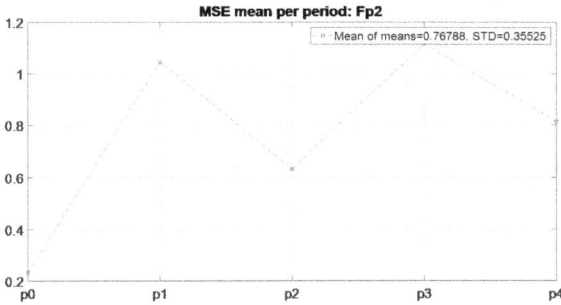

FIGURE 4.5: MSE mean of all MSE indices given in Figure 4.4. It is very easy to see the complexity of any period for any channel.

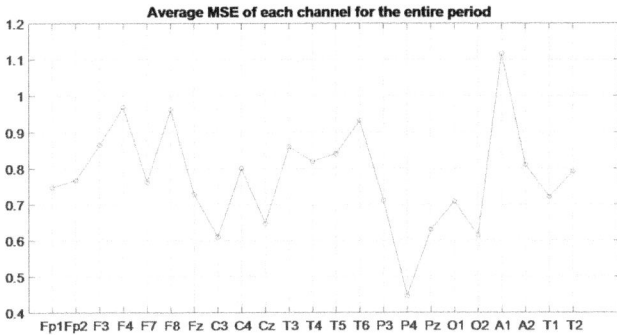

FIGURE 4.6: MSE averaged for all channels during the 52 minutes of the study. In this EEG, during all this time, the worst region (more seizures) was P4 as it can be seen above.

recorded for. In this form, suppose that we want to observe the entropy information contained in 30 minutes of time. One way is to create 30 slices of MSE (1 minute long each) and put them all together. Thus, curve 1 with a complexity plot for the first minute will be located next to the second plot corresponding to the following minute and so forth. All these slices next to each other define a complexity surface which is a function of time and sub sample rate τ. We named this new index/surface bivariate MSE or BMSE, i.e., BMSE=MSE(t,τ) [34]. The corresponding algorithm is described below. T_s is the EEG sample time and "n" is the number of slices (MSE curves) that will define the BMSE surface. Colon means step size in a vector.

Algorithm 2 Bivariate multiscale entropy (BMSE)

Input: $X = [X(1), X(2), \ldots, X(L)], \tau_{max}, \Delta\tau, Ts, n$.

Output: BMSE indices and a complexity plot BMSE=MSE(τ, MSE).

$L \leftarrow length(X)$
$t \leftarrow T_s * L$

Divide the whole time vector according to
for i=1 to n step size $\Delta\tau$ **do**

$$t(i) \leftarrow \left[\frac{(i-1)*T_s}{i} : \Delta\tau : \frac{i*T_s*L}{i} \right]$$

end for i

Compute the MSE slices for each t(i) and τ as follows:

for c=1 to n **do**

    Calculate MSE(c) with **Algorithm 1**

    BMSE(c) $\leftarrow$ MSE(c)

end for c

Plot a 3D graph: t and τ vs MSC(c), i.e., obtain BMSE(t,τ).

With the collection of BMSE surfaces, construct a film; i.e., a **complexity animation.**

Example 3. Running the later algorithm produces the surface shown in Figure 4.7. There, it can be seen that 15 minutes of EEG time is encompassed in a single graph. There are 180 MSE curves placed together. Each of them, contains the information of 5 seconds of EEG time (180×5 seconds = 900 seconds = 15 minutes). Notice that the lowest part of the surface is red (low complexity) and this behavior trends to go upwards gradually (regions yellow/green) up to high levels (in light blue). Similarly, for low values of τ, the sub sample signals looks like the original one and as tau increases, the signal is less alike to the original one. Combining the latter with the time-based behavior, the trend of this child's body is to recover (at least for this period of time). This can be deduced from the (slow) proclivity of the

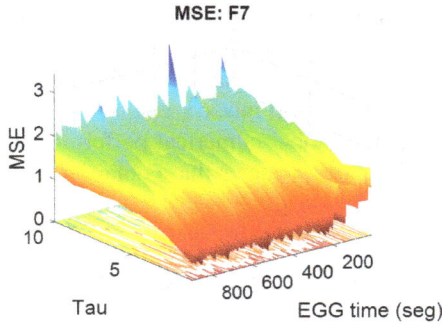

FIGURE 4.7: BMSE. Patient A, channel F7 for 15 minutes. Patterns of regularity in the EEG are reflected as red/orange portions at the bottom of the surface and non-regular (non/less convulsive trends in the EEG) are displayed as green/light blue sections at the higher parts.

surface to go from regularity (low values of entropy) to complexity (higher values of entropy).

4.2.15 Dynamic MSE index: dynamic complexity plots (complexity movie)

The surface illustrated before (Figure 4.7) is a single structure that covers 15 minutes of time. However, this idea can be extrapolated as it was done for MSE curves: at the moment, several MSE curves were computed for an arbitrary partition of time, and all together, defined a surface. Now, the analogy is: given a family of BMSE surfaces, let us define one of them for each partition of time. The product of this will be a group of BMSE surfaces comprising a certain interval of time. All of them will define a **movie** or **animation of complexity**. In this way, very long times can be encompassed easily.

Example 4. Nine BMSE plots of 6.7 seconds each are shown below. For instance, the upper right panel shows a clear seizure pattern in almost half of it but in the next one (for the coming 400 seconds) that pattern tend to dissipate. See patterns of colors. With the values on top of each panel a chart can be constructed showing only the BMSE indices linked to each lapse of time for this channel.

The above mentioned family of MSE parameters can be used to establish another measure associated to each entropy film. This parameter is referred to as ***dynamic bivariate multiscale entropy (DBMSE)***. Note that we also need to decide how many surfaces or frames we need in our film. The parameter for this will be nF. Moreover, this process can be practiced for all channels of the EEG whose results are quite beneficial because a lot of time is contained in a single point for all brain sections.

Example 5. The following set of DBMSE curves were computed for child C (image 4.2.15). From the average/standard deviations it can be seen that the worst period was the first one with an averaged DBMSE equal to 0.78356.

In similar fashion, it is possible to determine a single metric from each curve. The name of this space-time averaged DBMSE index is μ. This parameter was computed for three EEG periods (see left upper panel there).

Continuing this way, an overall index κ can be defined again by averaging all μ indices in order to obtain a global numerical performance for all the EEG periods by brain section. This is the parameter that contains information as completely as possible. See Algorithm 4 below [585], [587], [586].

4.2.16   Dynamic complexity parameters: DBMSE, μ, κ

Algorithm 3 computes DBMSE indices in order to plot them by period and brain zone. Figure 4.9 permits the observation of the entropy associated with each brain channel for several periods at the same time. Let us reflect that these graphs are very objective ways to display the neurological state of a patient for many periods. Moreover, it is possible to compare these collections of graphs among several patients. Evolution of similar diseases is now objectively comparable for parents and neurologists. Scrutinizing Figure 4.9 we realize that we can define another dynamic parameter for the whole brain (all channels), μ, as the average of these DBMSE indices. So, μ will show the entropy of the whole brain for a given period (or even periods!) of EEG time.

In this sense, the most condensed information will be encompassed by averaging all indices κ. Naming this new variable μ, will show the complexity associated to the whole brain for all periods of EEG time. Furthermore, these complexity numbers

---

Algorithm 3 Dynamic Bivariate Multiscale Entropy (DBMSE)

Input: $X = [X(1), X(2), \ldots, X(L)], \tau_{max}, \Delta\tau$, m, T_s, n, nF, num_chan.

Output: DBMSE indices and a DBMS surface.

$L \leftarrow length(X)$
$t \leftarrow T_s * L$

Divide the complete EEG time by the number of frames (BMSE surfaces) as
$tF \leftarrow t/nF$

Calculate DBMSE for all channels of the EEG.

for i=1 to num_chan **do**

        Compute BMSE(i) with Algorithm 2

        DBMSE(i) $\leftarrow$ mean(BMSE(i))

end for i

Plot DBMSE for each channel and for any period.

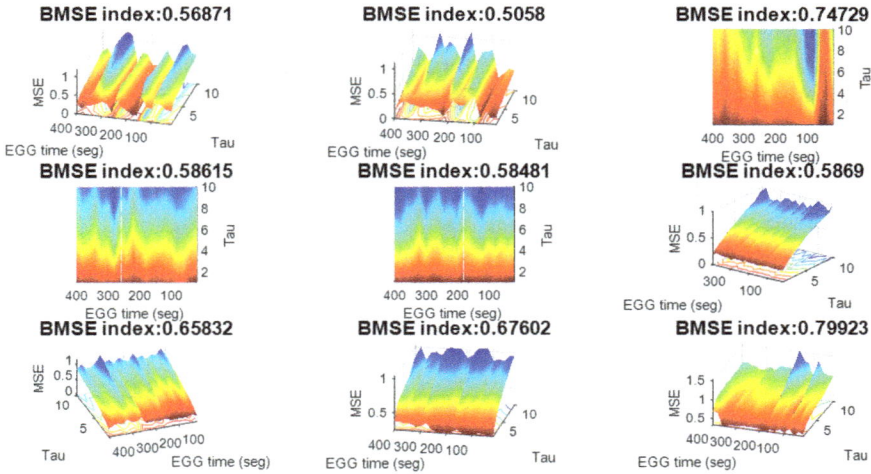

FIGURE 4.8: Frames of a **complexity movie**. Patient B, channel F7. EEG time consists of 400 seconds times 9 surfaces = 3600 seconds (1 hour) of EEG time. Although the film does not flatten the surfaces, this was done in this image in order to clarify the change in complexity with respect to time and τ. Observe the red/orange tones associated to low complexity states (see wavy patterns) and - in contrast- blue tones related to high complexity; improvement in seizures/conciousness. Nevertheless, notice that all BMSE indices are $BMSE < 1$, indicating predominance of seizures (as an average in a constant seizure-recuperation state) for each frame duration, 400 seconds.

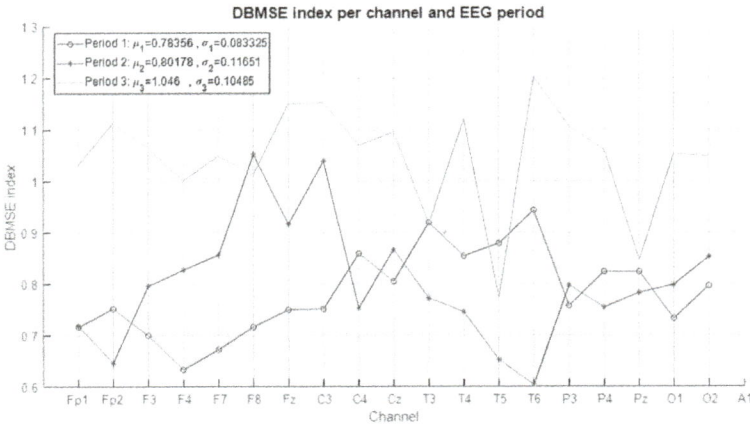

FIGURE 4.9: DBMSE plots by EEG period. In this way it is easy to observe the evolution of the disease with respect to time and brain portion.

permit making an objective comparison among many patients at the same time for all brain regions and for many EEG studies. See Algorithm 4 below.

In order to illustrate this, a table for all our involved subjects is provided below (Table 4.4). There, P stands for EEG period or study and S for subject; "w" means *worst*. NA means that a fourth period was not available for a patient. It is easy to identify the worst period/subject pair. It is easly identified that the most affected patient is child B and the healthiest is A. Observe also the standard deviation of this parameter.

We can complement this tabular information with the anticonvulsant drugs per patient (see Tables 4.1, 4.2, and 4.3).

TABLE 4.4: Complexity indices μ, κ and their standard deviation (σ) for all periods/subjects.

P/S	μ_A	σ_A	μ_B	σ_B	μ_C	σ_C	μ_D	σ_D	μ_E	σ_E
1	1.48	0.09	0.5	0.12 w	1.64	0.12	0.71	0.06 w	1.02	0.11
2	1.48	0.19 w	0.73	0.17	1.38	0.16	0.81	0.11	1.30	0.12
3	1.49	0.06	0.66	0.24	1.36	0.34 w	1.03	0.11	1.13	0.22
4	1.33	0.06	0.98	0.20	NA	NA	NA	NA	1.02	0.10
κ	**1.44**		**0.72**		**1.46**		**0.85**		**1.12**	

Algorithm 4 μ index, κ index

Input: $X = [X(1), X(2), \ldots, X(L)]$, τ_{max}, $\Delta\tau$, m, n, nF, num _chan, T_s.

Output: BMSE indices and a complexity plot BMSE=MSE(t, τ).

μ index: Averaged DBMSE by brain region
κ index: Averaged κ index

L $\leftarrow$ $length(X)$
t $\leftarrow$ $T_s * L$

Obtain DBMSE(i) with Algorithm 3
$\mu(i) \leftarrow$ average(DBMSE(i))
$\kappa(i) \leftarrow$ average($\mu(i)$)

Example 6. Running Algorithm 4 for all patients produces Table 4.4. From a simple analysis, it is deduced that patient B behaves the worst. This child has an associated entropy index $\kappa = 0.72$. This single number means that patient B, behaves majorly bad for all periods and for all brain regions because $\kappa < 1$. Obviousy, direct comparisons are immediatly done with the other subjects (normal subject E is not shown here but see details in [586]).

We undesrtand that we are offering our investigation as a useful resource for neurologists. Naturally, their diagnosis will depend also on the number of EEG studies, their duration, neuroimaging and blood tests among others.

4.3   Results: Entropy paths

Diagrams as the one given in Figure 4.2.15 were obtained for all subjects. From these pictures, it is possible to obtain the lowest value of entropy by EEG period. With that information, we illustrate here what an entropy path is (Figure 4.10). It is very useful to plot the trajectory of the most affected brain region on a 10–20 standard head diagram.

These entropy paths show the evolution of the worst case of a seizure per brain region per patient. Algorithm 5 computes these complexity paths according to the minimum value of DBMSE indices per EEG period and brain zone. Running this algorithm produces Figure 4.10. There the spatial complexity trajectories of the four subjects are illustrated. In addition, these pathways are listed next:

- Patient A: F8 → Fp2 → Fz → Cz.

- Patient B: F4 → Fp1 → P4 → T5.

- Patient C: F4 → T6 → T5 → T5.

- Patient D: T3 → F3 → C4 → C4.

Observe that in the case of patient A, the worst brain activity mainly moves inside the frontal lobe. This activity finishes in the central/central (Cz) zone of the brain. This result is in line with the clinical information of this patient where the focal lobe was identified as the main focus of this multifocal case. Patient B reflects the situation where the worst seizures (lowest enrtopies) move from one region to the other (and

---

Algorithm 5 Entropy paths

Input: num_periods.

Output: Entropy paths

for i=1 to num_periods **do**

       With Algorithm 3 determine DBMSE,

       DBMSE(i) ← min(DBMSE(num_periods)

       Identify Brain_zone(i) ← Zone_at(Min_DBMSE(i))

end for i

for j=1 to num_periods **do**

       With Algorithm 3, calculate min(DBMSE) per period and brain zone,

       Draw entropy paths on the 10–20 diagram

       Obtain κ from Algorithm 4

end for j

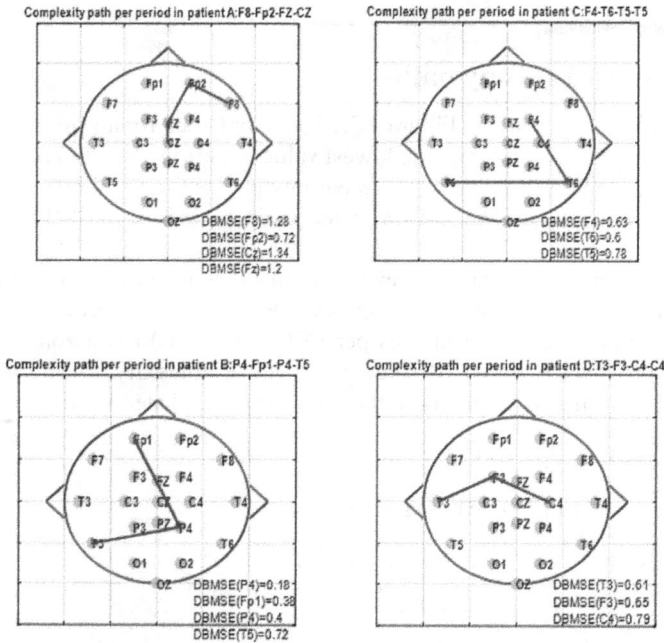

FIGURE 4.10: Entropy paths corresponding to the 4 patients of the study. It is possible to identify the path followed by seizures by region. DBMSE indices per region are also given to locate the worst among them as well.

with respect to their corresponding EEG period). In contrast, patient C, shows a more localized progress of the worst seizures. Finally, patient D is a sort of "mixed case" where the lowest parameters are associated to temporal-frontal zones and later, these discharges remain in C4. Proceeding like this, we can compare the evolution of these epileptic syndromes for multiple patients for all brain regions. These methods reflect space-time evolution for many patients at the same time in an objective way. Our results were also in line with clinical records.

Although the pictures shown in Figure 4.10 belong to very long term periods, these pathways can be obtained for short times.

Figure 4.11 illustrates a case of shorter EEG periods, where the DBMSE graph was obtained for periods 1, 2 and 3 with a duration of 5 minutes each. It is interesting to identify a minimum for the first period plot which occurs at F4. However, selecting a minimum for the second graph is remarkable because DMSE(T6) and DBMSE(Fp2) are almost equal. This event repeats for the third trace where DBMSE(T5) ≈ DBMSE(Pz). The latter means there are two complexity pathways that are almost numerically equivalent:

- Π_1: F4 → T6 → T5

- Π_2: F4 → Fp2 → T5

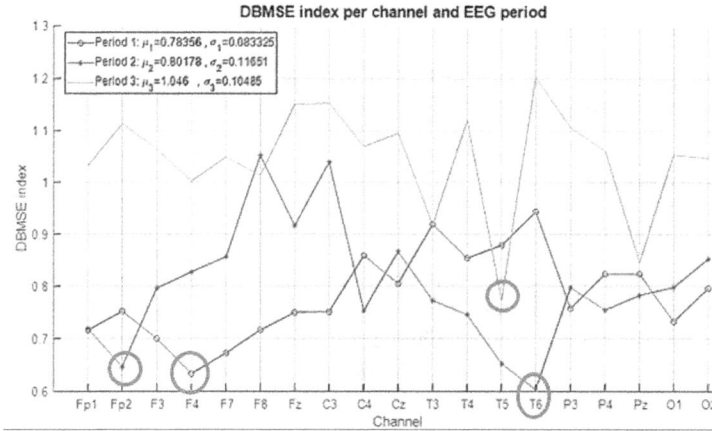

FIGURE 4.11: Minimum DBMSE indices per brain channel. Each period corresponds to 5 minutes of EEG time. Clearly, each curve has a minimum value which defines an entropy path: F4 → T6 → T5. However, notice that despite having these minimum numbers, there are other DBMSE that are numerically close to those minima. See Figure 4.12.

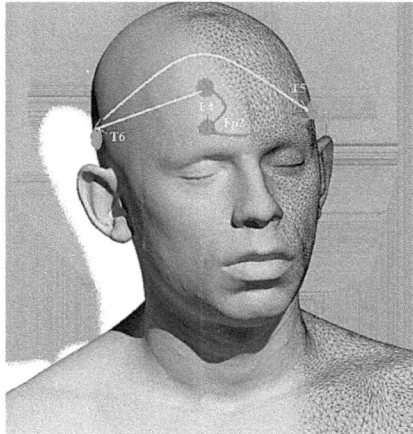

FIGURE 4.12: Consider Figure 4.11. There are two almost equivalent entropy trajectories: F4 → T6 → T5 and F4 → Fp2 → T5. This means that although the worst case is the first path, the second one is close to being like that. Observe the way seizures spread according to Sections 4.1.1, 4.1.2, 4.10.

The latter trajectories are illustrated in Figure 4.12. As mentioned before, the first 5 minutes of EEG time identifies a min(DBMSE) at F4. In the next period (second curve) we realize that DBMSE(T6) ≈ DBMSE(Fp2) and both ways finish at T5. We offer now a definition for this phenomenon. We will say that both trajectories are *almost equivalent* or that the complexity of both paths are almost equivalent, i.e., $\mathcal{C}(\Pi_1) \approx \mathcal{C}(\Pi_2)$.

Perceive that our MSE,BMSE, DBMSE, μ, κ indices, plots, and tables, objectively answer the questions established in the **Abstract** of this document.

4.4   Conclusions

Throughout this manuscript, the progress of a family of nonlinear statistics, known as complexity measures has been exposed together with graphical interpretations. These metrics and their associated graphs permit the comparison of the EEG studies of a single patient (from one period to the other) taking into account that in EE (epileptic encephalopathies) as in Doose and Lennox-Gastaut syndromes, many EEGs are collected through the patient's life. Moreover, the latter can be practiced with other patients in order to contrast information in an objective way. It is possible to find out which region/period was the best/worst by patient and compare and conclude among them. This fact answers the questions posed at the beginning of the document (Abstract), naturally answering parents' and physicians' inquiries.

5

Mobile and Home Electroencephalography in the Usual Environment of Children

Belinda Carrion* and Luis Felipe Herrera Padilla

5.1 History of telemetry in electroencephalograms (EEGs)

Telemetry can be defined as the automated measurement and transmission of data from a distant location via wireless transmission such as radio waves, cellular devices, or electrical currents. The data obtained is collected in an acquisition system where the results can be displayed. Among the major applications of telemetry is its use in health care for real-time patient monitoring. Employment of this technology is relevant for tracking bio-signals using tests such as the electrocardiogram (EKG), electroencephalogram (EEG) and electrooculography (EOG) [292, 210].

Neurophysiological studies such as EEG were only possible by monitoring the patient connected by wired cables inside a hospital. The usefulness of mobile or ambulatory EEG in patients with suspected seizures was recognized in the early 1970s [36]. In 1975, Ives and Woods showed that it was possible to aid the diagnosis of neurological disorders with the use of an in-home EEG. The devices to carry out the EEG consisted of four recording heads and 1/8-inch cassette tapes, with an on-head preamplifier to transcribe into tape and a video playback to record up to 24 hours [143].

Later in the 1980s, a prolonged (more than 24 hours) ambulatory EEG with portable devices became commercially available. Ives later on, transformed the 4-channel EEG to a 16-channel device. A new function was added where patients were allowed to push a recording button when they experienced any symptom related to their condition. The disadvantage was the short duration available to record only for 45 min/tape [143]. Operational features of the device were added such as: digital real time, automatic search of a specific time, 64 bits of memory and alpha numeric registry of channel gain. The apparatus allowed a higher spatial resolution in the mid-temporal and mid-frontal region, but still lacked full coverage in the posterior region [158].

In the early 90s, digital continuous recording of the EEG became possible using sixteen to thirty-two channels [36]. It was no longer mandatory to fit the recorder

School of Medicine and Health Sciences, Tecnologico de Monterrey, Monterrey, Mexico.
* Corresponding author: bca@tec.mx

to a portable computer to see online data. A Video recording system was added in order to monitor real time behaviour of the patient. Over the years, memory devices such as removable hard disks downsized increasing their capacity making it easier to record more than 24 hours of continuous monitoring [134].

Previously, EEG mobile devices required an instrumentation box placed on the belt and long wires that connected the recording device to the electrodes. Nowadays, these have transformed into a wearable electronic device that is wireless. The reduction in the length of the cables removed the interference created during motion, providing an upgraded data collection. In the 21st century, wireless transmission was introduced, and all the information accumulated was placed in a small box mounted on the head. Recently, the use of ambulatory EEG has emerged in high motion environments such as cycling and running which verifies the capability of full free movement capacity [84].

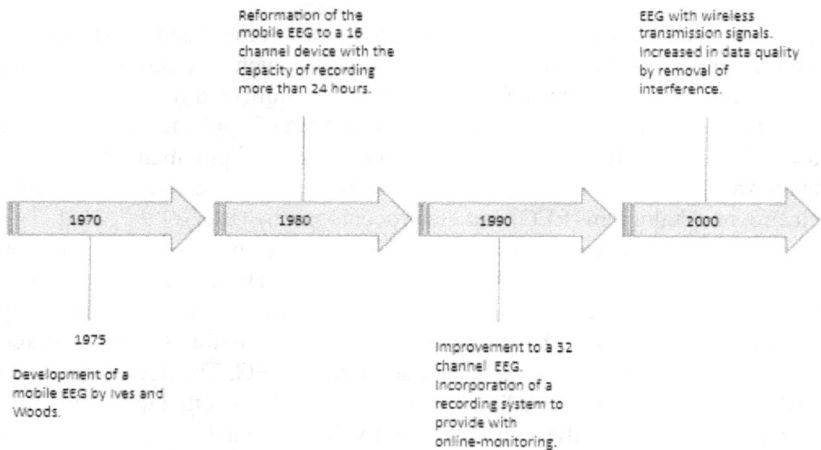

FIGURE 5.1: Evolution of mobile EEG since the 1970s until the 2000s.

5.2   Neurophysiological basis of EEG

An electroencephalogram (EEG) is a recording electrical communication activity of the brain. The electrical activity is registered by placing electrodes on the scalp with a conductive gel or paste, usually after preparing the scalp area by a light abrasion to reduce the impedance due to dead skin cells. The surface electrodes register electrical signals produced when brain cells send messages to each other. These signals are recorded by a machine and interpreted by an expert to identify unusual activity [529].

EEG uses the principle of difference in amplification, or recording voltage differences between different points using a pair of electrodes that compares one ac-

Signal acquisition	Wireless (Bluetooth)	Signal processing
Non invasive Electrodes	transmitter and receiver	Mobile device

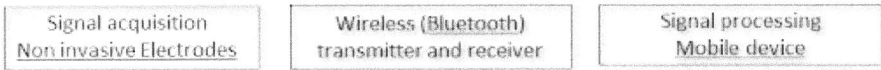

FIGURE 5.2: This diagram divides the EEG system into the signal acquisition, the transmission and processing that occurs in order to capture the bioelectrical activity of cortical neurons and translates it into differences of amplitude and voltage. Adapted from [305].

tive exploring electrode site with another neighboring or distant reference electrode [305].

The interpreter of brain electrical activity identifies deflection as explained. The direction of register deflection up and down represents activity from different electrodes. As such the voltage direction serves as shown in Figure 5.3.

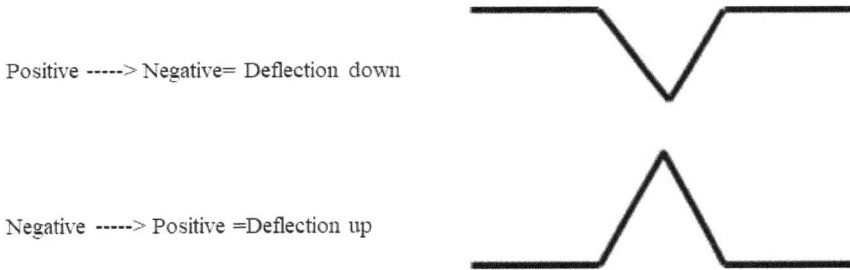

Positive -----> Negative= Deflection down

Negative -----> Positive =Deflection up

FIGURE 5.3: Figure of the register depending on the direction taken by the voltage.

Usually the purpose of the electrical registration of the cortical neurons activity fulfills two purposes: a) Defines an electrical basal rhythm across the surface of the brain b) Determines a focal disarranged circuitry that mainly reflects a damaged zone.

Observing the electrical basal rhythm of the neuronal activity gives information about the organization, continuity and discontinuity, symmetry, synchrony, amplitude, reactivity, and morphology of cortical circuitry. The frequencies of waves observed per second are related to brain maturity as can be observed in Figure 5.4.

Also regarding the wave amplitude generally the dominant cerebral hemisphere (the left side in right handers) can be considered "more active" [222].

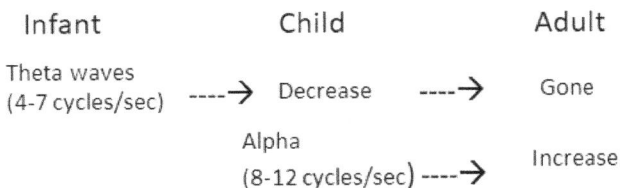

Infant	Child	Adult
Theta waves (4-7 cycles/sec) ----→	Decrease ----→	Gone
	Alpha (8-12 cycles/sec) ----→	Increase

FIGURE 5.4: Example of how basal rhythm changes through different stages of development.

Regarding a focal disarranged circuitry, the interpreter seeks to find out a phase reversal zone (Figure 5.5) or an equipotentiality (Figure 5.2). In the phase reversal zone an abrupt change is observed in a dipolar reading where the deflection direction sequence is as shown in Figure 5.5.

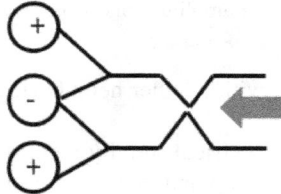

FIGURE 5.5: Phase reversal zone where the second electrode has a negative voltage compared to the first one.

In equipotentiality the voltage is abruptly increased over the basal level with a spread of voltage in nearby zones such as shown in Figure 5.6.

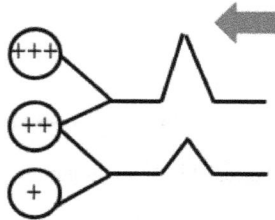

FIGURE 5.6: Abrupt increase in voltage from the first electrode with an excessive positive voltage.

5.3   Wireless and wearable devices for mobile EEG

Before introducing the subject of interest in this chapter it is important to clarify different interchangeable terms used such as: home EEG, ambulatory EEG, video EEG and mobile EEG.

Ambulatory EEG is synonymous to home EEG monitoring which is a test that measures and records electrical activity in the brain for up to 48 hours while your child is at home or school. This test uses a special recording unit that is slightly larger than a smartphone [459].

Mobile EEG also is synonymous to ambulatory EEG, but this term emphasizes the circumstances that are useful to monitor a patient's brain activity include walking outdoors with a wireless mobile EEG headset combined with a rucksack mounted PC [50].

Video EEG is used as a gold standard to diagnose nonepileptic seizures. During video-EEG monitoring, the patient wears an EEG transmitter connected to a wall outlet with a coaxial cable. Wall-mounted video cameras provide continuous behavioral observations [378].

The aims in research and development of mobile EEG is to provide lightweight sensors and shorter leads to prevent dragging or movement artifacts that may occur with prolonged home EEG monitoring [320]. Efforts have been made to develop wireless electrodes, bluetooth transmission and a mobile device for signal acquisition and processing.

5.3.1 Signal aquisition: Non invasive electrodes

There are two methods to hold electrodes in place over the scalp: wet and dry. Dry electrodes are much more difficult to secure to the participant and movement in relation to the participant's body occurs more readily. The wet method is the most reliable due to low impedance readings amd can be gel-based or saline. In this mounting an electrode paste is applied to improve the conductivity between the scalp and the electrode. Cotton or gauze often is placed over the electrode with cream to help hold everything in place. Collodion is sometimes applied onto the gauze placed over the electrode and is then dried [50].

The disadvantage of the wet method is that it requires a laborious process for application to the electrodes. That is why a self adhesive dry electrode has been developed and coupled with a specific high-impedance amplifier to record the brain electrical activity wirelessly.

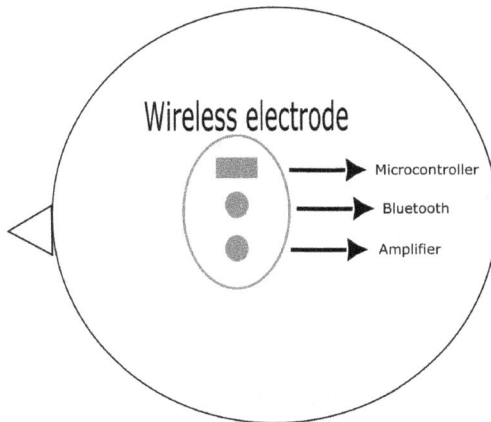

FIGURE 5.7: Diagram of how a wireless electrode can acquire the bioelectrical activity of cortical neurons and transmit its signal simultaneously.

One of the primary highlights of the mobile EEG is that the memory units are situated on the head, in contrast with past EEG units that regularly required an enormous and awkward instrumentation box to be worn on a belt with long cables to connect with the electrodes. This is a significantly favorable position compared to more established EEGs [85].

In order to allow mobility of the patient the amplifier can be mounted as shown previously to the head which has the disadvantage of increasing interference with head movement. Another option is mounted on the back placed in a rucksack [50].

5.3.2   Signal acquisition and registration

The most difficult thing about mobile EEG algorithms is to filter the noise caused by all the external factors that accompany a person in day to day life. A possible solution to this problem would be to use the ANOVA technique to define the best coefficient of the signal in the adaptation [300]. The quality of information collected by a mobile EEG is lower than a hospital or non-portable one, the possibility of having information on brain signals in real time and at low cost can be very useful for a better diagnosis [557].

5.3.3   Automated software for mobile EEG interpretation

Algorithms for detection of epileptiform transients have already been developed since the 1970s but are still not regularly used by EEG-reviewers. The difficulty in detecting epileptiform transients is that they have different morphologies that may be similar to artifacts and the absence of a common EEG database [36]. This is why it becomes necessary to create an automated software to detect EEG epileptiform abnormalities in prolonged EEG. This becomes more important for several reasons such as:

- Inexperienced physicians are prone to misunderstand the readings.

- It takes a lot of time for a person to analyze all the data gathered by the EEG (for a prolonged EEG, the recordings are usually 2 or 3 days long).

- The time spent by the physicians analyzing the data can be invested in other activities that cannot be done by automated software.

- In the near future, automated software could eliminate human error in interpretation.

5.3.4   Mobile EEG advantages and disadvantages

Among the advantages of mobile and home EEG is the absence of a need for the patient to be hospitalized, so no unnecessary time would be spent by the family members or the caregivers. The patient will be in a familiar and comfortable environment. Recording time will be for extended periods which would allow more data to be collected and if being recorded as a video, doctors can view patients remotely and continuously evaluate them. The waiting time to get a diagnosis would be drastically reduced [348].

TABLE 5.1: EEG mobile models.

Model	No. channels recorded	Type of electrodes	Data acquisition	Recording capacity	Video
ActiCHamp	64	Gel	SDRAM	24 Bits	No
Active Two	32	Gel	ActiView data acquisition	24 Bits	No
Ant	32 128	Gel	Remote web control, real time data access	32 Bits	No
Asalab	128	Gel	–	24 Bits	No
B-Alert	20	Conductive cream	Bluetooth, SD card	16 Bits	No
Brain Amp	28 120 156	Gel	–	16 Bits	No
Cognionics	10	Gel	MicroSD card	24 Bits	No
EPOC	14	Saline	USB receiver	14 Bits	No
Mindwave	1	Gel	Bluetooth Low Energy or Classic	16 Bits	No
MOBITA-W-32EEG	32	Water based	Flash Disk	16 GB	No
Nu Amps	32	Gel	USB interface to computer	22 Bits	No
Oldenburg Hybrid	14	Gel	–	14 Bits	–
Penso	8	Dry	Bluetooth to PC	16 Bits	No
Polymate AP216	3	Gel	PC/Compact Flash (2GB)	16 Bits	No
Profusion	32	Gel	–	16 Bits	Yes
Smarting	16 24	Gel	Bluetooth v2.1, PC or Smartphone	24 Bits	No
Safiro Ambulatory EEG System	Up to 32	–	Compact flash card	Up to 72 hours	No
Trackit MK3	21	–	Internal flash memory	Up to 96 hours	No
V-Amp	16	Dry	Recorder USB dongle blue	24 Bits	Yes
Varioport	10	–	SD card	16 Bits	No

Recordings during sleep are free of artifacts and almost 100% of the data is easily interpretable; on the contrary, daytime home recordings reduce interpretability due to facial muscle activity such as chewing [36].

The main concerns about mobile EEG are the risks of losing scalp electrode contacts that diminish signal quality, questionable reliability of EEG software interpretation. Since the development of high-input impedance amplifiers, very low skin-electrode impedances (b5 kΩ) seem to be unnecessary. Still, artifacts by body movements (walking, cycling), telephoning, tooth brushing and eating may hinder interpretation of the EEG signals [36].

Another disadvantage of home EEG might be the need for camera-video surveillance to be installed around the house of the patient, and to ensure that the patient's home would have the adequate broadband speed to have a reliable transmission. Also, with respect to the surveillance, if not enough cameras are available it will be difficult to watch the patient at all times unless he/she is restricted to certain areas. It has to be considered that not all patients have technically compatible houses to install all the surveillance gadgets. Another concern is the protection of the data generated. The data generated by the cameras should be properly encrypted and only be available for the analysis conducted in the hospital [158].

5.3.5   Mobile EEG for continuous epilepsy monitoring

Standardized EEG is limited to a brief recording time that spans between 20–30 minutes and the chance to detect an ictal (epileptic) or interictal abnormality is 30% compared to 70%. This is the main reason why prolonged EEG is needed and moreover recorded with wireless electrodes and mobile recording devices that can allow the likelihood of recording epileptiform activity [36].

The evolution of digital video-EEG monitoring has allowed the same EEG finding capabilities when performed either as ambulatory or as inpatient. In 1998 Liporace et al. found 15% seizure detection in ambulatory EEGs compared with none in the routine EEG [194].

Mobile EEG allows for prolonged recordings. Mobile EEG systems help to collect information on patients with epilepsy, which along with videos taken by the patient's parents is used by the doctor to reach a more accurate verdict on the patient's progress and avoid a misdiagnosis [84]. The evolution of digital video-EEG monitoring has allowed the same EEG findings capability when performed either as an ambulatory patient or as an inpatient at an epilepsy monitoring unit [194].

The International League Against Epilepsy recommends long term EEG monitoring where there is diagnostic uncertainty as to the diagnosis of epilepsy, in confirmed cases to classify the epilepsy syndrome, to quantify seizures or diurnal and circadian patterns, and to document the electro-clinical basis of seizures prior to surgery [158]. A review of the diagnostic yield to detect epileptiform abnormalities was done from 324 studies. Of these (68%) studies gave positive data: 36% showed interictal epileptiform discharges, 52% had epileptic events and 32% were normal. 22% of the studies changed the diagnosis and 29% refined the diagnosis by classifying the epilepsy as focal or generalised [158]. A recent study showed changes or refinement of the diagnosis after a long-term mobile EEG in 71% of patients referred for diagnostic clarification. Mobile EEG in the patient's home may be used for presurgical evaluation, syndrome classification or differentiation between epileptic and non-epileptic events [36].

5.3.6 Mobile EEG for nonepileptic attacks

The provisional diagnosis in paroxysmal disorders was epilepsy in 210 (65%), a non-epileptic diagnosis in 109 (35%) [158]. Psychogenic non-epileptic seizures (PNES) are episodic disturbances of reduced self-control associated with a range of motor, sensory and mental manifestations that resemble epileptic seizures, but are not caused by epileptic activity. They are also known as nonepileptic attacks [553].

Unfortunately it is common for nonepileptic attacks to be misdiagnosed and subsequent initiation of necessary antiepileptic drugs [423]. This is a reason to develop a proper EEG study to avoid misdiagnosis and wrong treatments. The International League Against Epilepsy recommends that video-EEG is the gold standard in the diagnosis of nonepileptic attacks [288].

80.2% patients benefited from undergoing ambulatory EEG after diagnosis of nonepileptic attacks in 50.5%. In three large studies it was shown that mobile EEG yields a diagnosis between 67.5 and 71.3% of nonepileptic attacks. The main benefit comes from capturing an event with no corresponding ictal change in the EEG [288].

5.3.7 Mobile EEG for neurodevelopmental screening

Neurodevelopmental disorders encompass a group of heterogeneous conditions that are defined by the Diagnostic and Statistical Manual of Mental Disorders, 5th edition as sharing the base characteristic of a delay in the development of one or more executive functions such as learning, social skills or intelligence. Conditions such as attention-deficit/hyperactivity disorder (ADHD), autism spectrum disorder (ASD) and language disorders are part of the group of neurodevelopmental disorders. These disorders frequently co-exist and have common clinical features such as learning, social and communication disabilities (DSM-V, APA 2013).

Event related potentiales (ERPs) are looked into in developmental disorders and have been proposed as biomarkers. ERPs have been described to reflect instances of attentional mechanisms, memory encoding and retrieval, response preparation and many more. ERPs are modulations of the EEG that are triggered by discrete events (either a particular stimulation or a movement) [550].

In the last three decades EEG studies seem as an ideal source for biomarkers since they provide a direct view of brain post-synaptic activity and have an excellent temporal resolution compared to other potential biomarkers such as Functional Magnetic Resonance Imaging (fMRI). Different biomarkers have been proposed during the years, such as the theta:beta ratio at vertex (Cz) for Attention Deficit Disorder (ADD), the role of brain symmetrization in language disorders, and the 'U shaped' profile for ASD. However most of these potential biomarkers haven't yet been sufficiently validated through rigorous clinical studies and meta-analysis [238].

The use of EEG biomarkers has also seen relative success in the field of ADHD. EEG technology has been used in ADHD for more than 80 years, when abnormal EEG rhythms at the fronto-central sensors were described in a group of children with hyperactive, impulsive and viable behavioral issues. These abnormalities were eventually formed into the theta-beta ratio (TBR) findings previously mentioned, where an EEG in an ADHD patient would show an elevated power of slow theta waves and/or a decreased power in fast beta waves at the fronto-central electrodes. This TBR seemed to have an excellent theoretical basis while providing significant sensitivity and specificity in aiding the diagnosis of ADHD, even so that an assistant diagnostic device rooted from this concept was approved by the FDA in 2013. However since then no study has been able to reliably prove the accuracy of the TBR, bringing controversy to the table. This EEG biomarker is yet to be proven clinically useful, either on child or adult patients, but developments in analytical and technological processes might aid EEG in providing some utility in the clinical sense in the near future. Another source of potential biomarkers for ADHD is the use of event-related potentials (ERPs). So far the most promising of these is the P3 ERP, which consists of a positive voltage deflection around 300 ms. This ERP is related to the evaluation of stimulus and response selection. P3 has been studied in multiple studies in adults, but the clinical meaning of this ERP is still unknown with the limited research around it [293].

In the case of Autism Spectrum Disorder (ASD), much of the EEG related research has been through the use of different analytical methods to produce distinct biomarkers that reflect the core EEG differences between a healthy control and a patient with ASD. Several studies have shown a possible lead into quantitative electroencephalography, an analysis method in which EEG signals are differentiated into their frequency bands through the use of Fourier Analysis. Fourier Analysis is a mathematical transformation that decomposes functions depending on space or time into functions depending on spatial or temporal frequency. In simpler terms, it is a type of analysis that allows the identification of patterns and cycles in a timed series of data. Several key EEG profiles have been identified through Fourier Analysis such as the U-shaped pattern, in which the resting-state EEG from patients with ASD show excessive power from delta and theta frequency bands while alpha frequency bands are diminished [546]. This pattern reflects a distinct rhythm maturation when compared to healthy subjects, in which the standard observation is an age-related decrease in delta and theta power and an overall increase of alpha power [217, 129].

Other profiles include the cerebral hemisphere asymmetry in regard to generalized power; ASD patients seem to have increased power in all frequency bands in the left hemisphere when compared to those in the right hemisphere, and discrepancies in the connectivity between different cerebral regions such as long-range underconnectivity compared to healthy subjects [546]. Some of these profiles can have a deep impact with clinical correlation, such as the epileptiform abnormalities which can be found in up to 61% of ASD patients. These patients with epileptiform abnormalities are more likely to have a severe form of the disorder and more intellectual disabilities compared to healthy subjects and ASD patients without these abnormalities [364]. Overall available data from EEG signal analysis has still failed to identify ASD patients with enough sensitivity and specificity to be clinically useful [195].

Another area in the world of neurodevelopmental disorders which has seen a development of the use of EEG technology has been language disorders. Language disorders EEG studies are relatively still in their infancy, but breakthroughs have been made. Studies have indicated that children with language disorders have a stronger global coherence in delta and beta oscillations, in other words a stronger global connection between both signals. In these children the role of brain asymmetry seems to be impaired as well, and the same studies have found that there is a higher synchrony between interhemispheric theta bands in the frontal regions of these children and they also show an increased interhemispheric coherence in all bands, making the case for an undeveloped brain asymmetry [182].

The research into EEG technologies and neurodevelopmental disorders have opened new areas of opportunity, some of which are still in their beginnings. The application of mobile EEGs in this field is yet to develop fully into research and clinical practice, but they have potential. Mobile EEGs can provide all the advantages of traditional EEGs while discarding some of their disadvantages in this population set [287].

5.4   Future trends towards mobility

Mobile EEG technologies have the potential to facilitate research and data-collection through the facilitation of large-scale studies not commonly seen in the traditional EEG field. Researchers and clinicians could soon have a new tool to live-test different variables such as real-world behaviours and treatment efficacy in these patients. While many forms of mobile EEG devices exist in the market there's still a lack of validation in the areas of signal quality, electrode density and headsets' comfort to fully integrate mobile EEG into large-scale data collection. Advances in the knowledge around mobile EEG technology are occurring rapidly, and soon these drawbacks might be overcome [287].

Wireless Brain Computer Interface (BCI) systems would provide users with more freedom of posture and movement so that they can perform their routine tasks in real-world environments. The front-end of a BCI (Brain computer interface) system can be integrated into a truly wearable device such as a baseball cap, a headband, or a pair of sunglasses to maximize portability and wearability [303].

Headset comfort and its development needs to integrate characteristics to fully acquire user acceptance in real life scenarios. The comfort of the subjects utilizing these devices is paramount for their successful use outside the lab. Losing the excess weight of the devices and improving their design comfort is part of the new trends evolving in the (BCI) scene [420].

The development of new BCI technologies must encompass a multidisciplinary approach. The combination of research by engineers, clinicians and software developers will overcome the challenges of improving BCI technologies. A recent study by Yadav et al. based on the trends and challenges of BCI technologies listed the following recommendations for successful progress of the application of these devices in both medical and non-medical fields. Some of the recommendations include [572]:

- Focus on the mental state of users rather than direct control of devices.

- Seamless integration with existing hardware and software.

- Standardization of BCI systems.

- Implementation of BCI technology outside the laboratory setting.

In order to develop their full potential, Mobile EEG technologies have been expanded into smartphone technologies. This could lead to a promising future for BCIs. EEG smartphone software applications such as the Smartphone Brain Scanner framework from MIT have shown relevant results in the use of EEG technologies in the smartphone setting. This framework provides data acquisition, data processing and applications in the mobile smartphone device through the use of external EEG hardware. Opportunities for smartphone EEG systems could propel the abundant use of these technologies providing valuable data for research in domains such as cognition, medical applications and social science research [502].

Clinical validation studies of similar smartphone application frameworks have been published in recent years. The technology still has ground to cover in order to be clinically useful; it could soon be a new way to introduce specialized neurological care in settings where standard EEG technologies are still largely unavailable [335]. In 2019 a group of researchers from America were able to enroll a group of children clinically diagnosed with epilepsy in West Africa in a remote EEG program with smartphone technology. The neurological researchers were able to document distinct epileptiform discharges in over 20 participants from a different continent, opening the chance for these low-income countries to receive specialized care from around the world [558].

Another scenario which will benefit from smartphone EEG technologies is home monitoring. Easy to use mobile devices could substantially improve the quality of home monitoring, with physicians being able to get real time information from their patients without setting up a clinic visit. EEG recordings coupled with a smartphone for signal processing has shown comparable quality with conventional EEG-systems while providing a low price and easy to use method [487].

The professionals involved in interpreting long EEG recordings to document seizures is costly and time consuming, that is why the tendency in modern EEG practice is to introduce computer-assisted technology as an automated mathematical analysis through Artificial Intelligence (AI) specifically machine learning [108].

Recent publications have shown the potential for machine learning in the analysis of EEG data. Artificial Intelligence (AI) has been shown to produce consistent results, such as in 2020 when a group of researchers were able to classify EEG emotion values through supervised AI learning. Their results showed that AI could correctly predict over 90% of the time which picture the participants were observing just by detecting emotional changes seen in the EEG [30].

Another group of researchers has developed machine learning algorithms designed to facilitate signal processing for the future use of motor-imagery-based BCIs, getting a step closer for humans to control robotic motor devices with just the power of their minds [15]. Machine learning algorithms have so far shown incredible results, and as this technology continues to develop the possibilities given to us by this field are progressively increasing.

5.5   Conclusion

Over the last decade the field of mobile EEGs has been advancing towards integrating this technology closer to our own bodies. Mobility research has been a key factor in this endeavor. The creation of "wearable" EEGs has been able to overcome the restrictions normally seen in laboratory or clinical setting machinery. Recent progress has deemed it possible to integrate this technology even further into our own bodies. This new technology is yet to be refined, and key aspects in signal acquisition have yet to be developed, but we might soon live in a world where wearable BCI devices are common practice for everyone. The main advantage in the new and discrete ways that are now being developed to take our own mobile EEGs anywhere is the ability to finally take the EEG out of the lab and use it in a real-world sense, where the application possibilities as of now seem endless.

6

Health: Human-Machine Interaction, Medical Robotics, Patient Rehabilitation

Pedro Ponce,* Erick Axel Martínez-Ríos, Juana Isabel Méndez, Arturo Molina and *Ricardo A Ramirez-Mendoza*

6.1 Introduction

Over the last couple of decades, there have been different types of approaches in which research has incorporated assistive technology to electric wheelchairs. For instance, the first documented prototype of an autonomous vehicle for people with restricted mobility is reported in the work of Madarasz et al. [417]. Despite the different types of approaches and navigation strategies that have been studied, like collision avoidance [415, 416, 486], path planning or wall following [174, 545], autonomous, and semi-autonomous control [401, 355, 125] along with the algorithms implemented to execute these strategies, there has been a common trend to steer the electric wheelchairs through unconventional hardware components with the main purpose of avoiding the use of a joystick. These methods include the use of voice commands, facial expressions (through computer vision), keypad, breath expulsion, head movements, switches input, or bio-potential signals such as electro-oculography and electromyography [443]. Nonetheless and regardless of the employed steering method, most of the proposals have only been concerned about user mobility, the interface or mechanisms to do so, and no other aspects like the health care or health monitoring of the patient. On the other hand, health monitoring systems incorporated into electric wheelchairs have used similar hardware setups like those used for the control methods mentioned above to measure the user's health state. For example, Lin Yang et al. [280] presented a mobile health care system for wheelchair users that integrates the use of electrocardiography, cushion pressure sensors, and an accelerometer to monitor the user's state while he is sitting on a mechanical wheelchair. Other works, as in [2], have incorporated similar architectures in their health care systems, but similar to the steering control methods, the scope of these proposals is limited to only health monitoring tasks. Figure 6.1 shows the overall Intelligent Electric Wheelchair architecture with each of the proposed subsystems. The voice, eye tracker, and head tracker signals send instructions to the HMI so that the wheelchair

School of Engineering and Sciences, Tecnologico de Monterrey, Mexico City, Mexico.
* Corresponding author: pedro.ponce@tec.mx

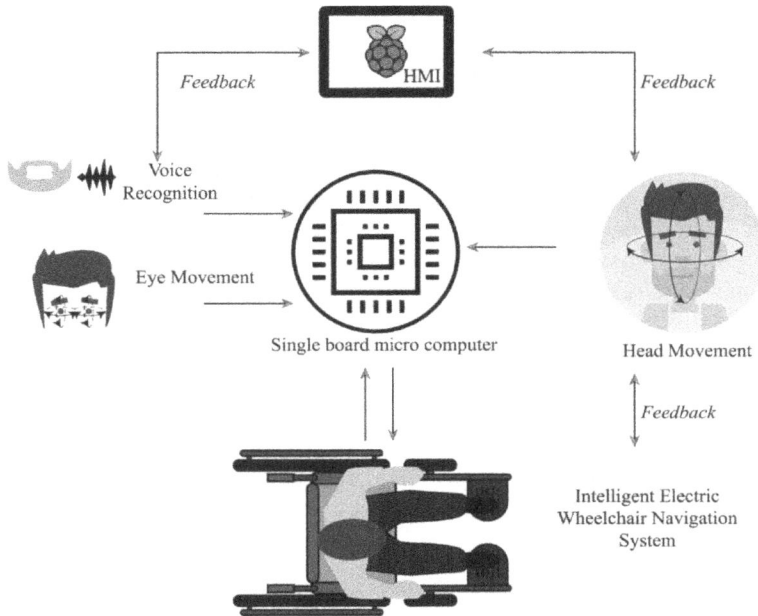

FIGURE 6.1: Intelligent Electric Wheelchair Architecture based on inputs genereted on HMI.

can follow the user's directions. The feedback between the individual, the interface, and the wheelchair promotes the system's stability. The HMI allows a user to have complete interaction with the system and vice versa.

6.2 Related work

This section presents the work related with electric wheelchairs as an assistive navigation device and as a health monitoring enablers for head movements, voice signal processing, and eye movements.

6.2.1 Electric wheelchair and assistive navigation devices

Most of the research regarding smart electric wheelchairs have been concerned with two significant areas. First, are the input interfaces to control the wheelchair without using the conventional steering methods like a joystick; second, in the navigation strategy used to assist the user during the steering of the device. For instance, one of the most common methods to control electric wheelchairs (EW) has been through bio-potentials such as electromyography (EMG) and electrooculography (EOG) [175]. The two methods have received particular attention in the literature for a long time. In [397], a literature review of the EMG control methods for power wheelchairs concludes that EMG techniques are recommended for both elderly and impaired users; moreover, for better performance in both pattern and non-pattern recognition, methods should be employed on the control commands. Electrooculography has picked up research interest since the studies of Barea et al. [44] employed EOG processing techniques to maneuver an electric wheelchair. Most recent proposals of EOG interfaces are presented in [90]. Whereas, other researchers use gestures to control EW through EMG and EOG [315] or combine electroencephalogram (EEG) with EOG signals to control EW [413]. Other techniques integrate computer vision systems into EW by image processing facial expressions and head inclinations to maneuver the chair [244, 419] or to monitor eye gaze through eye tracker devices [313]. Accordingly, any successful gaze-based system requires four elements [12]:

1. The system should recognize eye movements (recognition).

2. The user should not require training or use the eye in an unnatural way (no training).

3. The system should update and calibrate automatically based on the user and the situation (calibration).

4. The system should detect the user looking for an object or target, thinking or reading, among others (modes).

On the other hand, research has also been concerned with the EW navigation strategies to help the impaired user control it without making a great effort. One of the typical solutions uses a range sensor such as an infrared or ultrasonic sensor. The purpose of employing these sensors is to generate low-cost navigation assistance [190]. Some of the most common algorithms are obstacle avoidance, wall following, and doorway passing. Aside from before, EW prototype development has implemented artificial intelligence algorithms to enable an autonomous navigation strategy; for instance, Pires et al. [402] and Maatoug [248] developed fuzzy logic controllers for trajectory planning in their EW prototypes. Other navigation proposals use computer vision systems to enable an automated behavior of electric wheelchairs. Craciunescu et al. [314] used Convolutional Neural Networks to show a sophisticated computer vision architecture to detect floors and doors with high accuracy and speed and consequently generated a safe path to be followed.

Although EW commonly use biopotentials such as EMG, EOG, or EEG techniques to control EW, recently computer vision has picked up the attention of research since it is a non-invasive method that has generated better performance. One drawback of these types of interfaces is the fact that they require some specialized hardware to achieve good performance and reliability. On the other hand, navigation strategies have suffered for a similar effect in that research has opted to use image processing techniques to implement path planning and obstacle avoidance systems and to put aside less precise sensors like ultrasonic and infrared sensors.

6.2.2   Electric wheelchairs as health monitoring enablers

There has been an interest in the literature to enhance the capabilities of non-electrical or EW to improve the quality of life of impaired users. Some of the works have focused on developing posture monitoring and correction systems. Yang et al. [280] created a posture monitoring architecture through pressure sensors that emit alerts every time the user assumes a dangerous posture position. Similar work is presented by Ahmad et al. [229], in which an array of piezoresistive sensors was designed and constructed to detect irregular sitting postures effectively. Besides, Ma et al. [317] proposed a model to analyze the sitting behavior and body swings through a cushion by employing pressure and inertial sensors. Then, this author extracted statistical information from the cushion and conveyed recommendation exercises to the user. On the other hand, Arias et al. work [33] employs an unobtrusive multi-sensory system composed of force resistive sensors, a three-axis accelerometer, bal-listocardiography (BCG) sensors, and temperature and humidity sensors to prevent ulcer generation, heatstrokes and provide heart-monitoring capabilities. A similar study is presented in [39], where non-intrusive methods to measure electrocardio-graphy (ECG), photoplethysmography (PPG), and ballistocardiograph (BCG) were integrated into a chair. The development of health monitoring devices has also picked some interest in the literature, mainly due to the heart-related like ischemic heart dis-ease that people with restricted mobility are susceptible to acquire. For example, the study of Chow, Wang, and Chang et al. [102] shows the development of a real-time electrocardiography monitoring system with wireless transmission capabilities. An-other related investigation is shown by Dong-Kyoon Han et al. [206] in which an ECG system is coupled with BCG and kinetic sensors while a subject is moving or resting in a wheelchair. This data is transmitted to a remote medical server for further processing and analysis.

Another aspect has been the evaluation of fatigue while using wheelchairs. In [544], a neuro-fuzzy classification method is used to categorize the fatigue degree while using a wheelchair is presented. Likewise, Sonenblum et al. [493] describe a methodology to measure the use of manual wheelchairs movement effectively; the ar-chitecture uses a wheel mounted accelerometer to constantly measure the travel dis-tance and movement of the mechanical wheelchair and detect the long-term effects of steering it in health. Although there has not been a direct interest in measuring posture on wheelchairs through image processing, there have been some works that have tried to monitor posture with cameras. The use of computer vision for health applications has encountered a great variety of opportunities to provide solutions to domains like data visualization for image-guided diagnosis, operation rooms, ther-apy and surgery, assistance to motor-impaired users, and surveillance and support of the elderly. In the case of the assistance of motor-impaired users, some research has focused on generating gesture recognition algorithms to track hand and eye move-ments to control computer systems or electric wheelchairs. Computer vision has also served as a medium to monitor elderly people and create a smart sensor that can make motion tracking, activity modeling, and human-environment interaction mod-eling creating in this way a prompting mechanism that can notify doctors, caregivers, and families of the abnormal behavior in the monitored user. For instance, in [35–38] computer vision was employed in-home care and security monitoring mainly to detect emergencies in elderly and impaired people.

6.2.2.1 Head movements and health monitoring

Even though there are no health monitoring systems that use head movements through accelerometer sensors, the head is continuously related to other parts of the body. Thus, within the head, there are other activities to be monitored such as facial expressions, eye movements, tongue, and mouth behaviors. For instance, Cheng et al. [79] proposes the use of a Kinect to monitor the heart rate of the user by analyzing the pumped blood that circulates through the head and produces tiny oscillatory motion due to Newtonian mechanics. On the other hand, facial expression detection has also been of concern to identify patients [237]. Shamin et al. [316] proposes a cloud-based framework that recollects face images for later analysis and classification. Finally, in Nakajima et al. [249], a personalized recognition technique is proposed based on the space spectrum of the head top image for a biometric security system.

6.2.2.2 Voice signal processing for health monitoring

The literature has revealed that voice measurement and recording can provide a feedback on the user's health state. By studying features like the volume, intonation, rate of speech, and tone, it is possible to provide sensitive and valid measurements related to mental illness. Krzesimowski et al. [118] uses signal processing (time domain and frequency domain analysis) on voice recordings to monitor the hospitalization and rehabilitation process of patients that suffer from a stroke. A similar proposal is presented by Maharjan et al. [319], in which a smart speaker model is used to monitor the mental illness of the user; however, it avoids issues like security, privacy, and data storage. On the other hand, Mehta et al. [337] reports using an accelerometer placed on the neck for mobile voice monitoring. The signal bandwidth produced by the accelerator is measured to provide alerts to the user regarding his voice condition and, in this way, differentiates healthy and hyper-functional voice patterns.

6.2.2.3 EOG as health monitoring

As in the voice recording analysis, electrooculography has also been used to monitor patients' mental disorder diagnoses. For instance, Vidal reviews the potential of eye-tracking techniques, including EOG, which can be used for mental health monitoring based on psychological and clinical research. Some of the diseases that can be recognized through the study of eye movements are dyslexia, autism, Alzheimer's, drug consumption, and schizophrenia. Another application in which the EOG has been found useful is in the sleep-monitoring of patients. According to Sheng-Fu Liang et al. [8], electrooculography can be used for sleep monitoring of users, and in the same work it is mentioned that compared to electroencephalogram or polysomnogram recordings, EOG has the characteristic of being easy to place, and as a consequence, it can be controlled by the users without someone else's intervention. Additionally, the EOG technique has been used to classify common human emotions. Soundariya et al. [418], proposes a multiclass support vector machine algorithm to classify emotions like happiness, pleasure, wrath, sadness, and fear.

As a common trend in the monitoring devices integrated into the wheelchair prototypes shown above, it is possible to observe a trend in using non-invasive sensors or devices to analyze users' health status. The majority of the literature has taken advantage of the affordability of the force resistive sensors and accelerometers to detect lousy posture behaviors while sitting in the wheelchair. Nonetheless, the use of computer vision to detect bad posture behaviors has not been fully explored in smart wheelchair systems. Regarding the heart monitoring of the user, the most common techniques are ECG, PPG, and BCG, through non-invasive hardware and sensors.

6.2.3   Serious games as an assistive tool in HMI

Serious games (SGs) are the use of game elements within an educational purpose and ease learning in an entertaining environment by motivating the end-user. Talking about SGs means motivating students to learn new things either in an extrinsic or intrinsic manner [80]. Extrinsic motivation drives users through external rewards. In contrast, intrinsic motivation makes students achieve goals due to their inner, disinterested, and enjoyable motivation. Table 6.1 summarizes some intrinsic and extrinsic motivations collected by Chou et al. [103].

Besides, educational programs are created to engage productive learning environments in science, technology, engineering, and mathematics (STEM) domains [80]. Thus, it is relevant to know how to design a serious game for a specific purpose, for instance, teach the wheelchair users how to correctly use head movements, voice commands, and the eye-tracking. Thus, four conceptual pillars create a serious game design [142]:

- Player-centered design: End-users are involved throughout the design process to participate in the creative part of this pillar.

- Iterative development: The concept design, game design, and game development generate an interactive and incremental approach. During the design phase, the type of player and problem domain is identified and understood to propose the design

TABLE 6.1: Positive intrinsic and extrinsic motivations [103].

Positive Extrinsic Motivation	Positive Intrinsic Motivation
Narrative, elitism, humanity hero, higher meaning, points, badges, leaderboard, fixed action rewards, progress bar, quest lists, win prize, high-five, level up symphony, aura effect, step-by-step tutorial, challenges, rewards, virtual goods, build from scratch, collecting set, avatar	Beginners luck, free lunch, destiny child, co-creator, milestone unlock, evergreen mechanics, general's carrot, real-time control, chain combos, instant feedback, boosters, voluntary autonomy, choice perception, social invite/friending, social treasure/gifting, group quest, touting

concept. Then, the game design gathers the design concept to transform it into a full game. Finally, during the game development, the game is tested regarding its target, the technological side, and how much fun it is to provide the possible risk the game may have.

- Interdisciplinary Teamwork: All the elements involved participate in each aspect of the previous step to learn from each other's experience.

- Integration of Play and Learning: During this integration, the designers' background and expertise are equally integrated to ease the collaboration between all the involved parts.

Examples of serious games regarding the healthcare field are used to enhance learning, training, therapy, and rehabilitation practices. The aim is for experts to use serious games to aid people with heterogeneous characteristics as age, socioeconomic status, disabilities, skills, interests, and knowledge [534]. This chapter analyzes and presents the re-design architecture of an intelligent electric wheelchair and its Human-Machine Interfaces; hence, this interface uses the serious games to work as an assistive tool that teaches the users how to use the head movement, the voice command and eye-tracking accurately. Besides, the basis of this re-design relies on the preceding research works presented in [405, 436, 435] as part of the Innovation Product research group's projects of Tecnologico de Monterrey, Mexico City Campus.

Hence, the remaining chapter is organized as follows: Section 2 describes the material and methods using for the intelligent electric wheelchair. Section 3 presents the proposal for the voice, head, and eye command interface and the posture monitoring system. In consequence, Section 4 displays the results. Section 5 describes the scope of the prototype and discusses its advantages and disadvantages. Finally, Section 6 concludes and gives suggestions for future work.

6.3   Proposal

The EW's design executed the same interfaces and navigation system from [405, 436, 435] but through an open-source hardware and software to reduce its initial cost. Table 6.2 shows the characteristics and differences between the previous interfaces and biometrical control signals with the current re-design.

6.3.1   Assistive navigation device and posture monitoring system

This subsection depicts the methods and proposal for obstacle avoidance navigation systems and the posture monitoring systems.

TABLE 6.2: Characteristics and differences between the previous and current EW prototypes.

Elements	Previous [405, 436, 435]	EW Proposal
Characteristics	MATLAB® and LabVIEW were used in the previous iterations of the prototype for the interface and processing of the biometrical control signals.	C code and Python, which are open source programming languages with a great variety of resources that enable the quick development of applications.
Differences	The previous system was not accessible to all type of users due to the licenses.	The current system is affordable due to open source software.
Obstacle avoidance	X	X
Back posture		X
Head movement interface	X	X
Voice command interface	X	X
EOG interface		X

6.3.1.1 Obstacle avoidance navigation system

The semi-autonomous navigation system tried to prevent collisions with fixed or mobile obstacles while the user was operating one of the control interfaces. Therefore, a collision prevention strategy was implemented according to the direction that the user enters. In this case, the system had behavior, as shown in Figure 6.2. Thus, the assistive navigation control operated only when the user decided to move in one of the following directions: forward, backward, right, and left. Instead of implementing the whole fuzzy controller in an embedded system, as presented in [397], the implementation was simplified by generating a specific controller for each direction that the user could input.

In this case, four fuzzy navigation controllers for each of the four possible directions were designed using the Fuzzy Logic Toolbox from MATLAB. The input and output membership functions were based on [397]. The controller's surface was submitted to a polynomial regression to implement the fuzzy controller in a low-cost embedded platform; this process was similar to the one made for the Head Movement Interface. The generated polynomials area was programmed in the Atmega328p. The selected fuzzy logic controller was a Mamdani type controller [485, 345].

Since there was a complexity associated with the correct or precise implementation of the whole Fuzzy Logic Controller in a restricted embedded system, as is the case of an Atmega 328p, it was necessary to implement it in a different representation that helped to reduce the computational requirements. Therefore, the surface of the relationship between the FLC input and output relationship was submitted to a polynomial regression like the one done with the head movement interface (see Figure 6.3). In this case, the proposal used six PING ultrasonic sensors from Parallax to monitor the surroundings of the EW. The ultrasonic sensor range was limited to

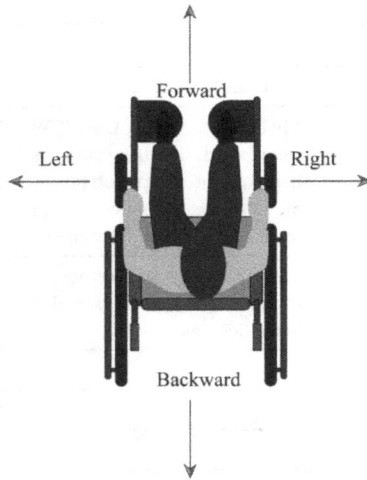

FIGURE 6.2: Intelligent Electric Wheelchair architecture using 4 basic commands.

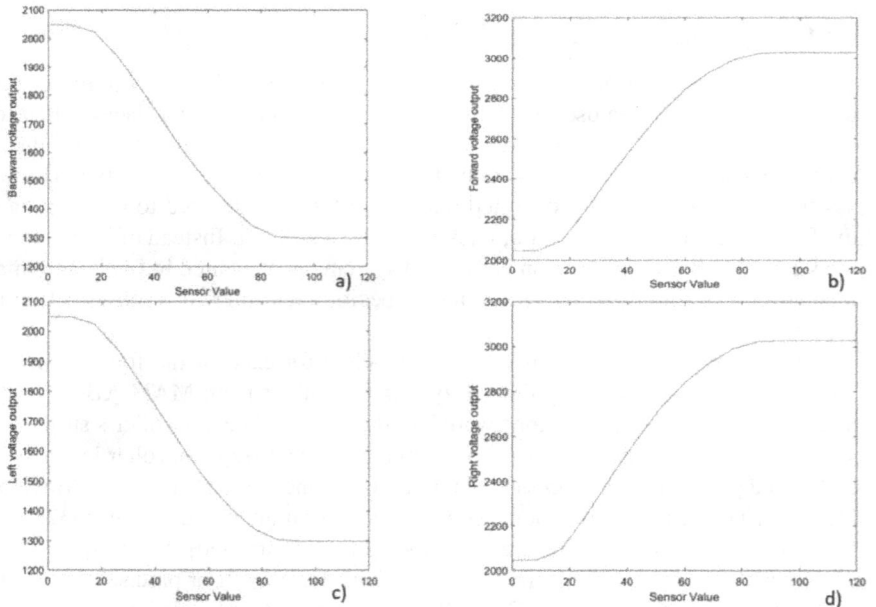

FIGURE 6.3: Back (a) and Forward (b) movement FLC surface and Right (c) and Left (d) FLC surface.

1.27 meters, which was the safety boundary of the electric wheelchair and, therefore, preventing a collision with a fixed or mobile obstacle.

6.3.1.2 Posture monitoring system

Some interfaces measure health conditions of the user; however, they require complex analysis and processing that may require some research on the specific topic. For instance, the voice and EOG recording analysis can determine the health state, leading to a more complex system that may require more intuition on the part of the user or caregiver. Nonetheless, according to the literature review, an area of interest and a health problem resulting from being in a chair all day due to restricted mobility is posture. Using this type of sensor prevents the use of invasive elements to monitor the user's posture behavior. The model of the Force Resistive Sensor was the FSR406. The circuit shown in Figure 6.4 sensed the changes in the resistance due to the pressure applied to the superficial area of the sensor. The Atmega2560 was the chosen microcontroller to perform the analog signal of the sensors. This microcontroller was selected due to the 16 analog to digital conversion channels that this microcontroller had, which were necessary to sample the distribution of the FRS sensors along with the seat and backrest of the electric wheelchair.

A bad posture is associated with health issues such as column problems or ulcers. Therefore, all the above generated this new proposal that monitors a bad sitting behavior in the wheelchair through force resistive sensors located in the backrest and cushion of the chair. The sampled frequency of the sensor was 10 Hz. Since this sensor was susceptible to high-frequency noise coming from the user pressure or mechanical vibration, it was necessary to apply a first-order low-pass filter that could wipe out the noise. Thus, a low pass filter had a cut off frequency of 1 Hz. The continuous transfer function was calculated using formula 6.1, leading to the next expression:

The binomial coefficient is defined by the next expression:

$$\frac{V_o}{V_i} = \frac{6.283}{s + 6.283} \tag{6.1}$$

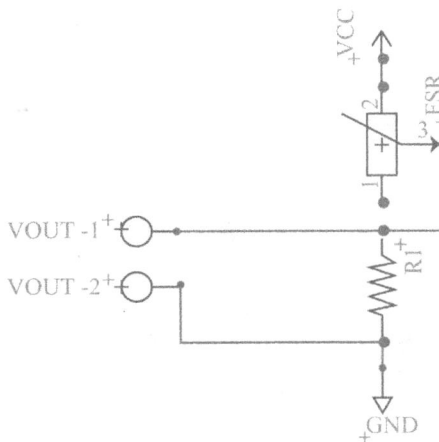

FIGURE 6.4: Force resistive sensor schematic.

A sampling frequency of 10 Hz to discretize the above transfer function was considered using formula 6.2 to map the continuous transfer function to the discrete domain. The above generated the next IIR filter:

$$\frac{Y}{X} = \frac{0.2391z + 0.2391}{z - 0.5219} \tag{6.2}$$

The difference equation programmed into the Atmega 2560 was presented as (see formula 6.3):

$$y(n) = (0.2391)x(n) + (0.2391)x(n-1) + (0.5219)y(n-1) \tag{6.3}$$

where y(n) was the current filter output, x(n) represented the actual filter input coming from the ADC of the microcontroller, x(n-1) represented one previous input value of the ADC; whereas, y(n-1) was the previous output value of the IIR filter. The rate of one of the timers was configured to the interrupt mode to generate fixed sampling and getting samples from the analog channel in equal intervals. Five resistive force sensors were placed on the EW, as seen in Figure 6.5. Three (F1, F2, F3) were placed at the top of the EW backrest, while two (F4, F5) were placed in the back part of the seat. F4 and F5 were used to measure the presence of a user in the EW with the correct seatbelt adjustment and to maintain a 90° neutral pelvis. Besides, any user must use the seatbelt of the wheelchair to prevent accidents while operating the system. The F3, F2, F1 sensors were in the top section of the backrest to measure if a user is not having a good sitting posture and to prevent sacral sitting.

Figure 6.6 shows the plot data from the five resistive sensors while a user is sitting in the electric wheelchair. Therefore, with that data, it was possible to monitor the column behavior based on the information gathered from the force resistive sensors placed on the back of the electric wheelchair. Moreover, there was a decrease in the ADC value sample, indicating that less pressure was applied to the surface of the force resistor sensor related to a possible curvature in the column. The values of the F1, F2, and F3 sensors must have had a reading value between 700 and 800 and if the sampled value was below 700, it indicated a sacral sitting posture that could damage the column and pelvis of the user in the long term.

Figure 6.7 shows the scatter data from the force resistive sensors F1, F2, and F3 divided into three classes based on the degree of sacral sitting posture. In this case,

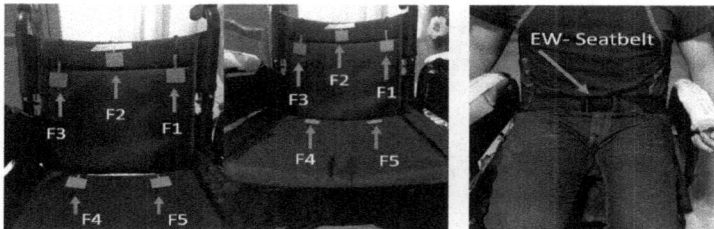

FIGURE 6.5: Force resistive sensors deployment in the seat and backrest of the electric wheelchair.

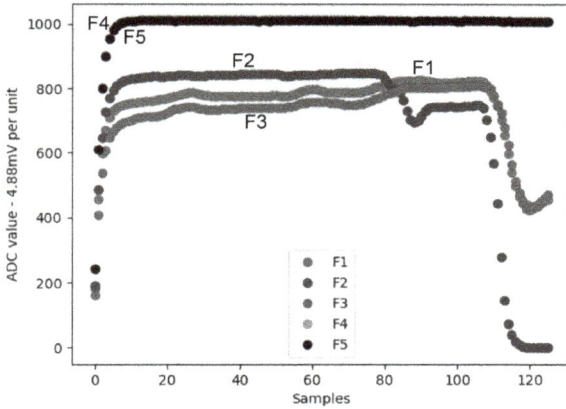

FIGURE 6.6: Data plotting of the force resistive sensors.

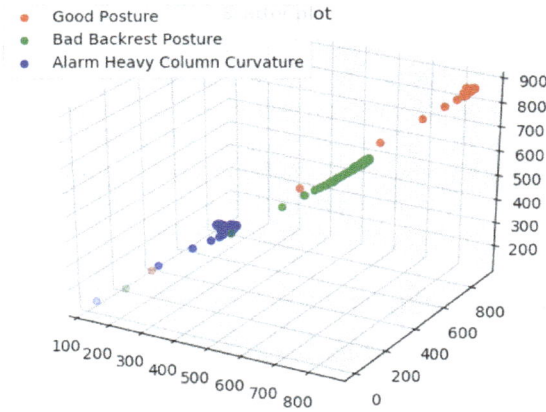

FIGURE 6.7: Scatter plot of the force resistive sensors.

the degree of curvature was labeled as "Good Posture", "Bad Back Posture", and "Alarm, Heavy Column Curvature". Three discriminant functions were calculated using Linear Discriminant Analysis (LDA) to classify this scatter data as in the EOG interface classification section of the present chapter. For this case, the x feature vector was expressed as (see 6.4):

$$x = [F1, F2, F3] \tag{6.4}$$

where F1, F2, and F3 were the ADC values of the FRS sampled by the microcontroller. On the other hand, the coefficients and the discriminant function using LDA for each class are shown below (see 6.5):

$$W1 = \begin{vmatrix} 0.05429692 \\ 0.26909971 \\ 0.0184828 \\ b1 = 146.64478674 \\ Z_1(x) = x^T W_1 - b1 \end{vmatrix}$$

$$W2 = \begin{vmatrix} 0.47038235 \\ -0.19446742 \\ -0.12106328 \\ b2 = 117.87310456 \\ Z_2(x) = x^T W_2 - b2 \end{vmatrix} \tag{6.5}$$

$$W3 = \begin{vmatrix} -0.23445684 \\ -0.24746657 \\ 0.53028575 \\ b3 = 85.75582631 \\ Z_3(x) = x^T W_3 - b3 \end{vmatrix}$$

With this new addition, the intelligent electric wheelchair not only helped steer it but also monitored certain health issues related to a bad sitting posture. Figure 11 presents the new system prototype. The wheelchair was a Powerchair model from Power Car. This wheelchair model was also more affordable than the previous prototype's EW. The analog input of the joystick is replaced from digital to analog converters with an output voltage between 0V to 5V to control the wheelchair through the proposed interfaces, as previously established in the head movement interface section.

6.3.2   Health monitoring enablers

This subsection presents the methods and proposal for the head movement, voice command, and EOG interfaces.

6.3.2.1   Head movement interface

Most of the research regarding smart EW have been concerned with two significant areas. First, there are the input interfaces to control the wheelchair without the use of the conventional steering methods like a joystick; second, the navigation strategy assists the user in steering the device. For instance, one of the most common methods to control electric wheelchairs (EW) has been through bio-potentials such as electromyography (EMG) and electrooculography (EOG) [175]. The head movement interface components used an accelerometer (MEMSIC 2125), an Atmega328p, 0 to 5 V digital to analog converter (DAC), and a Raspberry PI 4 Model B with a Linux based operating system. The model of the DAC is an MCP4725. The I2C serial communication protocol controlled the DACs. Since two DACs were used to substitute the voltage levels of the joystick of the electric wheelchair, it was necessary to assign a different address for each of the integrated devices on the I2C bus. For this prototype, a Raspberry Pi 4 Model B plus was used as the central processor. One crucial aspect to consider was that the Raspberry Pi requires a power supply of 5V and 3A, and a voltage regulator capable of supplying at least 15W is fundamental to the whole system operation. Consequently, a portable power bank with an 18W energy supply was selected. The microcontroller calculated the accelerometer's tilt in the 'x' and 'y' directions to control the wheelchair through the head movements. Based on the calculated tilt, a fuzzy logic controller assigned the wheelchair direction. Lotfi A. Zadeh proposed the fuzzy logic in his seminal paper on fuzzy sets in 1965 [580]. Fuzzy logic controllers (FLC) produced a non-linear relation between their input and output by using membership functions that represent the degree in which a linguistic variable belongs to a class between the ranges from 0 to 1, and linguistic rules usually expressed as if_then_ statements. Since then, fuzzy logic controllers had been used in a variety of applications like video cameras, air conditioners, and the automotive industry. Thus, the FLC considered the fuzzification stage, rules evaluation, and defuzzification stage [406]. Taking these characteristics into account, a FLC was designed to execute the head movement interface algorithm. The above led to the surface of the Sugeno fuzzy logic controller for the wheelchair's x and y directions (Figure 6.8). Following, which the surface of the input and output relationship of the calculated fuzzy controller was subdued to a polynomial regression. In this case, to assure that the obtained model explained all the variability of the surface, a square R major to 0.90 was obtained. Consequently, a third-order polynomial for both directions was used. The obtained polynomial equations were programmed in the Atmega 328 microcontroller for both directions (X, Y). The output value was sent through the UART serial communication protocol to the microcomputer.

The output value was sent through the UART serial communication protocol to the microcomputer. A Python 3 based Graphical User Interface (GUI) was developed to allow the driver to visualize the direction of the wheelchair and the values of the accelerometer.

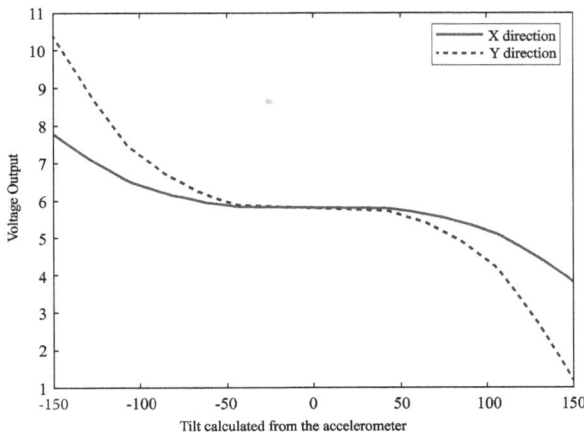

FIGURE 6.8: Fuzzy logic surface for the x and y output based on a Sugeno Fuzzy Logic Controller.

6.3.2.2 Voice command interface

The system used the Raspberry PI 4 and a USB microphone to implement a voice recognition application based on Python. In this case, the Speech Recognition module of Python was used along with the Sphinx API. The advantage of using the Sphinx API is that it is an open-source speech recognition model that does not require an online connection, unlike other APIs like the Google API, Microsoft Bing, or IBM speech to text models. Sphinx's problem was that the model was not accurate all the time, so the number of words the model needs to search for was restricted. For this case, five keywords were declared corresponding to the control directions possible for performing with the wheelchair; in other words, Left, Right, Forward, Back, and Stop were the voice control commands.

6.3.2.3 EOG interface

For the electrooculography (EOG) interface, the hardware set-up employed an amplification and pre-processing circuit to filter out the noise. The EOG signal was an electrophysiological technique used for sensing the bio-potential generated between the retina and the cornea and not from the muscles located around that eye. This signal was seldom deterministic even for the same person in a different environment since it was affected by factors such as luminance, head movements, eyeball, and eyelid movements. Other sources of noise during the measurement of the EOG were the skin resistance, electrode slippage, or wrong electrode placement. Due to the above, a well-designed signal conditioning system was required to counterweight the non-deterministic behavior of this biopotential. According to the Standard for Clinical Electro-oculography from the International Society for Clinical Electrophysiology of Vision (ISCEV), the frequency range of the EOG was located within DC 0 Hz to 30 Hz; nonetheless, due to the baseline drift to which this biopotential was susceptible, sometimes the bandwidth of the signal was suggested to be measured within the 0.05 Hz to 30 Hz range. Hence, it was crucial to filter out the signal in the specific bandwidth of interest. To the above, the first stage of the EOG acquisition circuit was the instrumentation amplifier. The selected instrumentation amplifier was an AD620N. This first stage was for amplifying the small EOG signal that has an amplitude of around 3500 µV. Since the EOG single was susceptible to low-frequency noise commonly known as baseline, it was necessary to add a decoupling stage for these low-frequency signals. For this purpose, a second-order high pass filter with a cut-off frequency of 0.05 Hz was added to the proposed circuit. Then to remove the high-frequency noise a 30 Hz, low pass filter was added. This filter also serves as an anti-aliasing filter for the analog to digital conversion needed to process the signal in the microcomputer. Finally, a buffer amplifier was added to the circuit, and the voltage output was sent to the digital to analog conversion channel of the Atmega 328p. Since it was important to minimize space and components that can consume both power and space from the electric wheelchair, it was relevant to use low power consumption components. For this purpose, the OP27GP operational amplifier and AD620 instrumentation amplifier fulfilled that requirement. Also, to avoid using a bipolar power supply or the use of a two-series battery in the system, a 5V charge pump with a negative output voltage was used to supply the operational amplifiers. The charge pump used for this purpose was the LM2662, a switched capacitor voltage converter recommended for operational amplifiers, power supplies, and medical instruments.

The microcontroller's conversion from an analog to a digital unit was employed with a 10-bit resolution to sample the signal with the Atmega 328p. Then, the Nyquist theorem was considered; thus, a sampling frequency of at least 60 Hz was required as the bandwidth of the electrooculography signal is around 0.05 Hz to 30 Hz. Besides, a sampled frequency of 250 Hz required an oversampling that avoids aliasing problems in the sampled data. Nevertheless, since two analog channels needed to be measured for vertical and horizontal movements, the 250 Hz sampled rate was duplicated, leading to a sampled frequency of 500 Hz. An interrupt service routine of an 8-bit timer of the microcontroller was used to assure a fixed sample rate. To further remove the high-frequency noise, a second-order infinite impulse response (IIR) digital filter was designed and implemented in the Atmega 328p, considering the previous adjusted 500 Hz sampling rate with a cut off frequency of 12 Hz. The continuous low pass filter was first calculated to design the IIR, leading to the next transfer function (see 6.6):

$$\frac{V_o}{V_i} = \frac{5685}{s^2 + 150.8s + 5685} \tag{6.6}$$

With the above transfer function, it was possible to map it to the discrete domain through the use of the bilinear transform or Tustin method. By considering a sampling rate of 2 ms, the discrete transfer function of the continuous transfer function was (see 6.7):

$$\frac{V_o}{V_i} = \frac{0.004916z^2 + 0.009831z + 0.004916}{z^2 - 1.72z + 0.7392} \tag{6.7}$$

The above discrete transfer function was programmed in the microcontroller by expressing it as a difference equation (see 6.8):

$$y(n) = 0.004916x(n) + 0.009831x(n-1) + 0.004916x(n-2) + 1.72y(n-1) - 0.7392y(n-2), \tag{6.8}$$

where y(n) is the current filter output, x(n) represents the actual filter input coming from the ADC of the microcontroller, x(n-1) and x(n-2) represent previous input values of the ADC. Whereas y(n-1) and y(n-2) were the previous output values of the IIR filter. Since the IIR filter output values depend on values from the same output from the past, it had a recursive nature in the programming of the differential equation and the performance of the filter in the frequency domain. The sampled and filtered data was sent through a serial communication protocol; for this purpose, the UART communication protocol was used. The data was later processed in the microcomputer to perform a feature extraction analysis and model classification to create an automated eye movement recognition system that controls the wheelchair's direction based on the eye movements. To generate the classification model's data set, different samples of right, left, up, down, and blink movements of the eye were recorded. In this case, three features were extracted from the EOG signal for each of the recorded movements. First, a 2.048s window was recorded, from this window, the root mean square, the average rectified value, and the distance between the minimum and max peak values of the signal were used as features to classify the eye movements. Ten samples with their corresponding features were recorded to be used as data to create a classification model. LDA was selected as the classification technique to generate the classification model. As its name suggests, it generated a linear decision boundary between two classes by finding the projection in space that maximizes the variance between classes and minimize the variance within each class. The reasons for choosing this technique were that it was applied to multi-classification problems, comparing it with the logistic regression that becomes unstable. Thus, it gave good results with fewer samples, as it was stable even though the data was far apart. One characteristic of LDA was the assumption that the observations or predictors from each class came from a normal distribution with a particular class mean and common variance [235]. Therefore, it was assumed that the selected features have the above characteristics. The discriminant function was obtained using the next equation in matrix representation by assuming more than one predictor in the observations (see 6.9):

$$\delta_k(x) = x^T \Sigma^{-1} \mu_k - \frac{1}{2}\mu_k^T \Sigma^{-1} \mu_k + log\ (\pi_k), \qquad (6.9)$$

where k represented the class to be analyzed, which assumed values from 1 to N classes. μ was the mean of the k class, Σ was a covariance matrix between the k classes, π was the class membership probability of the k class, and x was the new observation to classify. The discriminant function needed to be calculated for each of the K classes; therefore, to determine if a new observation x corresponded to a specific k class, the value of the discriminant function evaluated for an x observation generated the highest value in the k discriminant function. The features for the classification of the eye movement were time domain. These features were the average rectified value; the root mean squares and the distance from the highest peak of the signal to the lowest peak of the signal.

6.3.3   Serious games

Table 6.3 describes the positive intrinsic and extrinsic motivation considered for the three interfaces based on [103]. These elements were chosen to teach the users how to use the electric wheelchair, in which the positive intrinsic motivation was proposed to motivate the users to feel included within their environment. In contrast, the extrinsic motivation was displayed, so the user actively learned the activities.

TABLE 6.3: Positive intrinsic and extrinsic motivations used in the interfaces.

Positive Extrinsic Motivation	Positive Intrinsic Motivation
Narrative, points, badges, progress bar, level up symphony, step-by-step tutorial, challenges, rewards, virtual goods, collecting set, avatar.	Beginners luck, real-time control, instant feedback, choice perception.

6.4 Results

With this new development and design of the human-machine interfaces developed for the electric wheelchair prototype, it is possible to considerably reduce the development time and cost of the previous iterations of the intelligent electric wheelchair compared to what is shown in [175, 397, 44].

The three interfaces considering a SG structure are shown in Figure 6.9. All the interfaces display the directions, the initiated modality, the tips which can be read or heard by the user, and the profile which the end-user can access through the voice command "Access to my profile". The distribution of the interfaces is as follows: in the upper part the three modalities are displayed, the center part depicts the directions with a central white bar that shows the direction performed of the wheelchair, in the bottom part the buttons to the exit interface, the tips and the profile are displayed. Figure 6.9(a) displays the interface in the educational form; hence, the user can learn how to use the three modalities of the interface: voice, head, and eye. Figure 6.9(b) shows the home page; Figure 6.9(c) presents the voice navigation, in which the center white bar displays in a statement the direction of movement. For instance, if the word is not recognized correctly, the program will display an "I do not understand" message, and the wheelchair will not move. Figure 6.9(d) presents head navigation and Figure 6.9(e) presents eye navigation. When the direction is activated, one of the circles is highlighted; otherwise, the four direction circles are highlighted, meaning that there is no movement in action.

Figure 6.10 depicts the instrumentation of the distance sensor, head interface, electrooculography interface, electrodes, and touch display with the Raspberry Pi. Moreover, this prototype does not require the use of specialized software and hardware like MATLAB and LabVIEW due to its use of C codes for the microcontroller devices and Python for the data processing with the Raspberry Pi. Therefore, it helps making the product feasible, reproducible, and scalable into a commercial product in the midterm.

6.4.1 Intelligent electric wheelchair in a COVID-19 context

With the actual global pandemic COVID-19, there are more than 40.6 million cases [113]. For instance, in Mexico, there are more than 850 thousand cases, with more than 200 thousand active cases [223]. Therefore, health monitoring can help identify, track, and forecast outbreaks, or enable communication during periods of reduced human-to-human physical contact. [302].

For instance, by linking the intelligent wheelchair with other products at home, the users can pay more attention to their family and interact with friends while the wheelchair is monitoring their health. An example of interaction is proposed in [354], wherein the elderly users are monitored through Alexa and cameras (gesture and voice) to track their mood to avoid depression. For instance, Figure 6.11 displays a proposal of the home screen considering the interaction with Alexa and watching the tips in videos.

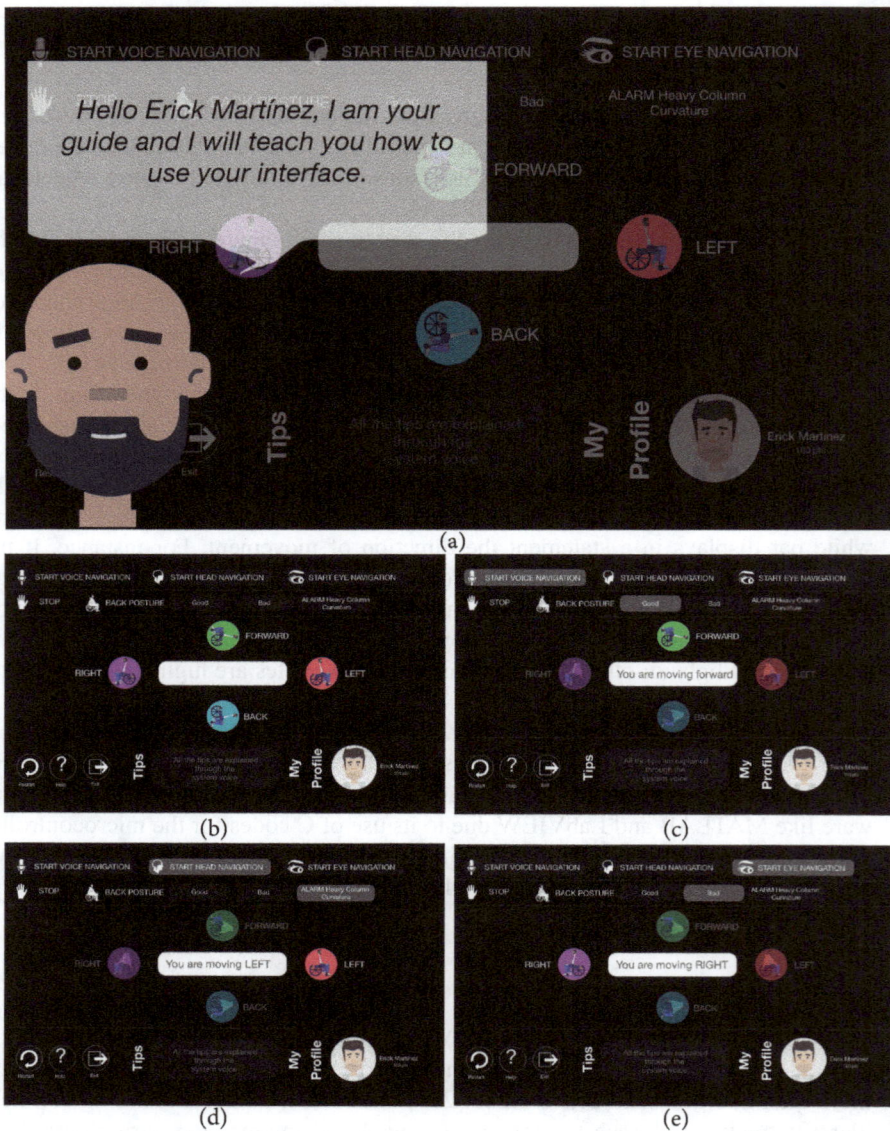

FIGURE 6.9: Interfaces with a SG structure for the voice command, head, and eye navigation. (a) General Interface with a guided help. (b) General interface. (c) Voice navigation interface. (d) Head navigation interface. (e) Eye navigation interface.

Therefore, electric wheelchairs represent a suitable instrument by taking advantage of the interfaces to socially connect the users with the family and other end-users and to promote a social interaction.

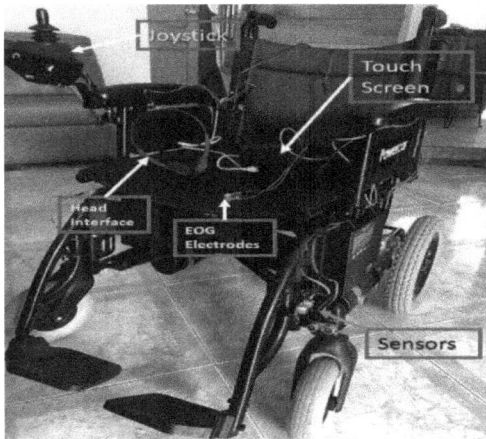

FIGURE 6.10: Electric wheelchair components distribution.

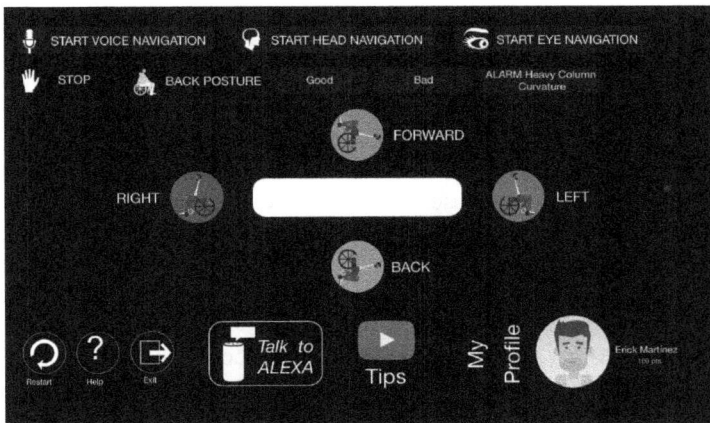

FIGURE 6.11: Interface proposal considering the interaction with Alexa within a Smart Home.

6.5 Conclusions

In this chapter, biometrics signals such as voice commands, head, and eye movements are used to provide information on the user-health condition to redesign an intelligent electric wheelchair. A SG interface is designed to teach users how to use this type of chair through friendly interfaces. This redesign simplifies a fuzzy logic navigation controller for obstacle avoidance to be embedded in a low-cost processor. Hence, three human-machine interfaces (voice commands, head, and eye movements) are proposed to steer a conventional electric wheelchair. Besides, a new posture monitoring system is implemented using non-invasive elements such as FRS. This monitoring system seeks to improve posture conditions when the end user is sitting in the chair and his/her posture is incorrect. Furthermore, more health monitoring systems can be added to the prototype, like electrocardiography and photoplethysmography.

This chapter analyzes and redesigns an intelligent electric wheelchair and three interfaces for the voice, head, and eye movements based on preceding research works proposed in [52–54]. The goal of this project is to design a friendly electric wheelchair which includes a HMI in order to be driven by the end-user. Besides, the HMI is running a gamification system that helps to learn the characteristics of the electric wheelchair. Therefore, this new electric wheelchair prototype's architecture implemented in this chapter uses electronic hardware developed from zero and new artificial intelligence algorithms with open-source embedded systems for data acquisition and processing. Besides, the microcontrollers and microprocessors use C code and Python to allow accessibility and reduce license costs of paid software. For the assistive navigation device, the prototype uses ultrasonic sensors that monitor the electric wheelchair's surroundings and is limited to 1.27 meters for safe boundaries to prevent collisions. Regarding the posture monitoring system, five resistive force sensors are placed on the electric wheelchair, and the use of a seatbelt is mandatory. Besides, the interfaces display a "Good Posture", "Bad Back Posture", and "Alarm, Heavy Column Curvature". In this proposal, the health monitoring enablers considered a USART serial communication protocol for the microcomputer for head movements. The voice system uses the Sphinx API; however, it is not as feasible as other APIs like Google, Bing, or IBM speech, so few voice control commands were declared. In the case of the eye movement interface, the pre-processing circuit was designed using a few low cost hardware components to reduce the space needed to place the sensor, and the computational requirements due to the type of learning model used to classify the eye movements and also for implementation in the hardware and software of the algorithm.

Regarding serious game elements within interfaces, the proposal considered the use of more extrinsic motivation than intrinsic motivation to motivate the user to learn and take advantage of the wheelchair. One main advantage of this new design is the use of a LCD and the absence of a whole computer system or laptop for data processing and human-machine interaction as in previous iterations, making the previous prototypes unsuitable for commercial use and clinical protocol testing environments. Moreover, this new prototype added the column posture recognition that previous iterations did not consider. FRS were used in the backrest of the chair, proving that this method is feasible for implementation as it requires low computational features and is non-invasive for the user. The use of more sophisticated techniques like computer vision for health monitoring was discarded in this approach of the new wheelchair architecture due to privacy and security reasons related to the user acceptance of the prototype. Besides, the use of image processing requires more complex processing, which could increase the cost of the prototype. The interfaces could be updated with further research by providing tailored interfaces based on the user requirements and tailored serious games strategies that engage the user and take more advantage of the EW. Moreover, this prototype could be connected within a Smart home architecture, in which the users can interact with the home or voice systems such as Alexa if they want to another relevant aspect is the new disease and the new systems and prototypes needed to ensure user safety. For instance, with the EW, users could track social distance accurately with distance sensors. Even the user's health information can work for the health care sector where doctors can monitor users' health and detect if the user is being compromised and could be infected, for instance, with the COVID-19 virus.

6.6 Glossary

Assistive technology: Any device, equipment, software program, or product system that increases, maintains, or improves the functional capabilities of persons with disabilities or the elderly sector.

Electric wheelchair: Power chair or motorized wheelchair.

EEG: Electroencephalogram, is a test that uses tiny metal disks (electrodes) attached to your scalp to detect electrical activity in your brain.

EMG: Electromyography, is a form of electrodiagnostic medicine to determine and document the electrical activity produced by skeletal muscles.

EOG: Electrooculography, is a technique for calculating the corneo-retinal standing potential that occurs between the front and the back of the human eye.

Fuzzy logic: It is a branch of Artificial Intelligence that allows a computer to analyze information from the real world on a scale between false and true.

Human Machine Interfaces: Dashboard, layout, or canvas that links the end-user to a machine, device, or system.

Non-invasive sensors: Devices that do not penetrate, inject, or incise the body.

Serious Games: Use of game elements within an educational purpose and ease learning in an entertaining environment by motivating the end-user.

7

APSoC-Based Implementation of an EEG Classifier using Chaotic Descriptors

Hugo G Gonzalez-Hernandez,[1],* David Antonio-Torres,[1] Walther Carballo-Hernandez[2]
and *Ricardo A Ramirez-Mendoza[3]*

7.1 Introduction

The World Health Organization, WHO, describes epilepsy as a chronic brain disease characterized by recurring seizures that affects people worldwide. Seizures are brief episodes of muscle contractions that could affect some part of the body (tonic-clonic seizure) or all of it (generalized tonic-clonic seizure), which sometimes are accompanied by loss of consciousness and control of bowel or bladder functions [152]. In Mexico, epilepsy is prevalent in 10 to 20 people out of every 1000, leading to the estimate that at least a million people suffer from an epilepsy variant. In Mexico, unfortunately, there exist many developing zones and non-urbanized or remote areas where, statistically, the prevalence of epilepsy is expected to be higher than urbanized areas [70].

Pattern recognition on electroencephalogram signals (EEG) is a complex process that consumes an enormous amount of analysis time, even for professionals in the area. With the proper use of mathematical tools for the description of time series, the processing of such signals has been made viable to be integrated in machine learning systems, specifically, for classification purposes [83]. Many methods have been proposed to detect epilepsy through EEG signals. Wang et al. report the simulation of a model described in Verilog of a *lifting-based Discrete Wavelet Transform* with an accuracy of 95% [548]. Selvathi et al. report the MATLAB® modeling and FPGA (Field Programmable Gate Array) programming of an epilepsy detector based on the count of amplitudes and determination of the frequency of digitized signals and compared with signals defined as normal, however, the percentage of accuracy is not reported [461]. Harender and Sherma computed statistical descriptors such as mean power, standard deviation and absolute average from the decomposition of EEG signals with the *Discrete Wavelet Transform*. Their Matlab models yielded an

---

[1] School of Engineering and Sciences, Tecnologico de Monterrey, Puebla, Mexico.

[2] Institut Pascal Université Clermont Auvergne, Aubière, France.

[3] School of Engineering and Sciences, Tecnologico de Monterrey, Monterrey, Mexico.

* Corresponding author: hgonz@tec.mx

accuracy close to 100% using public databases. The performance of their model in an embedded system has not yet reported [211].

This article proposes the use of chaotic descriptors, such as dimension correlation, Lyapunov exponent and Hurst exponent, to train support vector machines (SVM). In turn, the SVMs are used as classifiers to determine the presence of tonic-clonic seizures in EEG signals. The mathematical modeling has been conducted with MATLAB and Simulink and the paradigm of model-based design [329] has been followed for the purpose of automatically generating the programming code of the embedded system.

The paper is organized as follows: Section 7.2 discusses the EEG public database used in our work. Section 7.3 describes how the characteristics of the signals used by the chaotic descriptors are extracted. Section 7.4 provides a brief introduction to SVMs. Section 7.5 describes the embedded classifier, while Section 7.6 discusses the results obtained with such a classifier. Finally, Section 7.7 draws some conclusions on the results using the proposed classifier.

7.2   Basis for EEG measurements

For the present work, three data sets of the public EEG database of the University of Bonn, available online, have been chosen for this work [373], the data sets are designated as Z, F and S and consist of one hundred segments with a duration of 23.6 s, obtained from an EEG according to the 10–20 standard for the electrode pads placement system. The segments of the Z set are of five healthy subjects in relaxing state with open eyes. The segments of the F and S sets result from the intracranial measurement of the epileptogenic zone of five patients, the former without a seizure and the latter during a tonic-clonic seizure [27]. The signals that showed artifacts (strong eye movements in Z and pathological activity in F and S) were removed by visual inspection by an expert. After a 12-bit analog-to-digital conversion, the selected data were captured by a data acquisition computer with a sampling frequency of 173.61 Hz. Subsequently, the data were filtered by a Butterworth pass-band filter with a band pass of 0.5–40 Hz, which is large enough to cover Delta and Gamma brain bands. The problem at hand consist in classifying the state in which the patient is and not if she/he is with open eyes and out of an epilepsy seizure, which is indicated by the O set, or if the seizure occurs in the lobe opposite to the epileptological zone, indicated by the N set. Some signals of the five classes are shown in Figure 7.1.

7.3   Feature extraction and chaotic descriptors

The first step in the classification process is the feature extraction from data. This process is carried out because a great amount of data within the measurements is to be classified, and it is of vital importance that the selection of these features is such the that data to be considered for the classification will be reduced in size, leading to

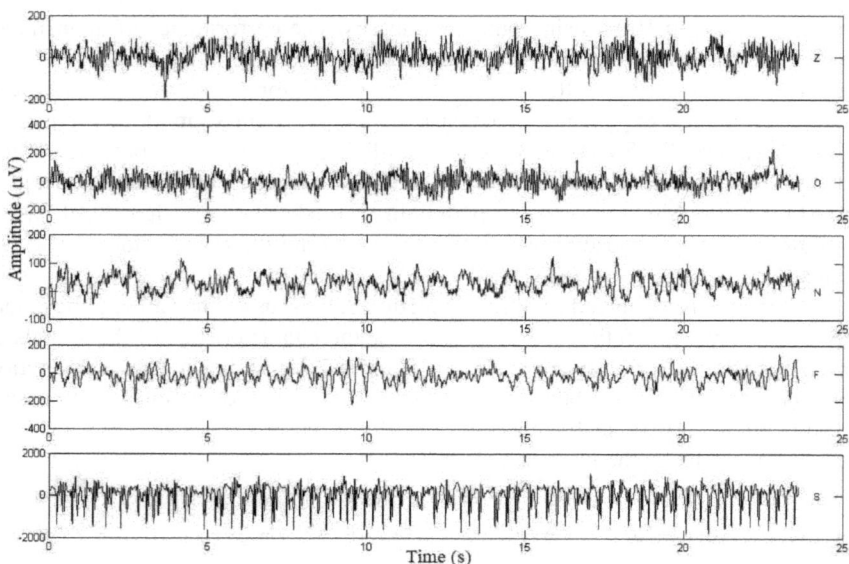

FIGURE 7.1: Samples of the EEG database of the University of Bonn.

a more compact feature space, i.e., a descriptor space in which a point in this space gives information about the chaocity of the signal, is called a chaotic descriptor. For this experiment, three chaotic descriptors were extracted from 100 EEG segments for classes Z, F and S, then a 3-dimensional descriptor space was constructed. In what follows, a brief description of the methods to compute the chaotic descriptors is depicted.

7.3.1   Attractor reconstruction

The extraction of certain features requires a previous processing involving the reconstruction of the dynamics of the system in the state space from a time series. We use the so-called *delayed coordinates* technique [256], by which m-dimensional vectors are created manipulating the scalar time series x and obtaining delayed versions of the original time series:

$$y(n) = [x(n), x(n+\tau), \ldots, x(n+(m-1)\tau)] \tag{7.1}$$

where $\tau \in \mathcal{N}$ denotes the time spacing in multiples of the sampling period between time series data used as coordinates for each vector, and m denotes the dimension of the reconstructed vectors. Therefore, we have two parameters to be determined for the reconstsruction, the *time delay* τ, and the embedding dimension m, it is common to use the *Average Mutual Information (AMI)* for τ and the percentage of false nearest neighbors *False Nearest Neighbors (FNN)* for m.

7.3.2 Average Mutual Information (AMI)

The average mutual information between a couple of continuous variables continuas A and B with probability function $f(a,b)$ is an efficient method for the estimation of the delay time τ. Before describing the mutual information formally, a few considerations should be made. First, if the value of τ is small, coordinates $x(n)$ and $x(n+\tau)$ will not be independent enough; and second, if τ is too big, any connection between these coordinates will be numerically subject to be random. In [171] and [3] the suggestion is to select τ based on a fundamental aspect of chaos phenomena: the information generation. The concept of average mutual information is based upon Shannon's information concept. Let us consider two measurements $x(n)$ and $x(n+\tau)$, the mutual information between these measurements is the quantity learned by the measurement $x(n)$ about measurement $x(n+\tau)$, such that AMI is given by [3]:

$$AMI(\tau) \quad = \quad \sum_{x(n),x(n+\tau)} P[x(n),x(n+\tau)] \qquad (7.2)$$

$$\log_2 \left\{ \frac{P[x(n),x(n+\tau)]}{P[x(n)]P[x(n+\tau)]} \right\}$$

where $P(\cdot,\cdot)$ is the joint probability density and $P(\cdot)$ is the individual probability density. A straightforward prescription to determine if measurements $x(n)$ and $x(n+\tau)$ are independent enough to be considered as coordinates of the reconstructed vector $y(n)$ is to choose τ where the first minimum of $AMI(\tau)$ occurs.

7.3.3 False Nearest Neighbors (FNN)

In order to obtain the embedding dimension m, we consider the FNN technique. The fundamental idea to find m is that if the embedding dimension is big, then a couple of points which appear to be near in the reconstructed space could be far from each other in a larger dimension. These points are described as False Nearest Neighbors. Explicitly, the criterion for the identification of false neighbor is as follows; consider the vector [429]:

$$y(k) = [x(k),x(k+\tau),x(k+2\tau),\dots,x(k+(m-1)\tau)] \qquad (7.3)$$

The nearest neighbor is determined by finding the vector that minimizes the euclidian norm $R_n = \|y(n)-y(k)\|$. Now consider each one of those vectors in an embedding dimension $m+1$,

$$y(n) \quad = \quad [x(n),x(n+\tau),x(n+2\tau),\dots,x(n+(m-1)\tau),x(n+m\tau)] \quad (7.4)$$
$$y(k) \quad = \quad [x(k),x(k+\tau),x(k+2\tau),\dots,x(k+(m-1)\tau),x(k+m\tau)]$$

In the embedding dimension $m+1$, these vectors are separated by a distance $R'_n = \|y(n)'-y(k)'\|$. We use a couple of criteria to identify a false neighbor [256], Criterion 1 is (7.5):

$$\sqrt{(R'_n - R^2_n)/R^2_n} = \frac{|x(n+m\tau) - x(k+m\tau)|}{R_n} > R_{TOL} \qquad (7.5)$$

where R_{TOL} is an adimensional tolerance. For our case, we experimentally have chosen $R_{TOL} = 50$. Criterion 2 is (7.6):

$$R'_n/R_A > A_{TOL} \qquad (7.6)$$

The last criterion is introduced to compensate criterion 1 due to the possibility of having scattered portions of the attractor. Here R_A is a measurement of the size of the attractor for which the standard deviation of the data is used [256]. If criterion 1 or criterion 2 is satisfied, then $y(n)$ is considered a false nearest neighbor (FNN) of $y(k)$. The next step is to find the total number of FNN and the percentage of false neighbors with respect to all neighbors. A suitable embedding dimension is such that the percentage of false neighbors is close to zero.

7.3.4   Correlation dimension (D_g)

The idea behind the well-known algorithm proposed in [192] is to find the fractal correlation dimension to construct a function $C(\varepsilon)$, which is the probability for two arbitrary points in the reconstructed trajectory to be inside a D-dimensional ball of radius ε. This function, called *correlation sum* is normalized such that when ε is big enough, $C(\varepsilon) = 1$. Assuming that N points are taken from the trajectory in the state space and avoiding duplicity [494]:

$$C(\varepsilon) = \frac{2}{N(N-1)} \sum_{j=1}^{N} \sum_{i=j+1}^{N} \Theta(\varepsilon - \varepsilon_{ij}) \qquad (7.7)$$

where Θ is the Heaviside function and ε is the spatial separation between a couple of points labeled i and j, typically given by the euclidian norm. The logarithmic plot of $C(\varepsilon)$ vs ε should be approximately a straight line with the slope being the correlation dimension at the limit for small ε and big N.

$$D_g = \lim_{r \to 0} \lim_{N \to \infty} \frac{d \log(C(\varepsilon))}{d \log \varepsilon} \qquad (7.8)$$

7.3.5   Largest Lyapunov exponent (λ)

Lyapunov exponents are the divergence rates of two close trajectories within an attractor with respect to time. A necessary but not sufficient condition for a system to be chaotic is that the largest Lyapunov exponent (LLE) should be positive. In [438] a widely used algorithm is depicted for computing the LLE from a time series. The first step in the method is the reconstruction of the state space, then the closest neighbor is determined for each embedding vector. The LLE is estimated as the average divergence rate of the neighbors. Assuming a separation determined by LLE then, at time t, the average divergence will be $d(t) \backsim Ce^{\lambda t}$, where C normalizes the initial separation. The natural logarithm to both sides of the equation leads to:

$$\ln d(t) \backsim \ln C + \lambda t \tag{7.9}$$

Then a set of parallel lines for different embedding dimensions is obtained, and LLE (λ) can be estimated using a standard least square procedure of the average slope of all embedded vectors.

7.3.6 Hurst exponent: H

Hursts exponent quantifies the correlation between points of a time series with a re-scaled range R/σ. The equation 7.10 describes the finite variance of a time series.

$$R/\sigma = \left(\frac{\pi n}{2}\right)^{\frac{1}{2}} \propto n^H \tag{7.10}$$

where R is tha range of cummulative sums given by the difference between the maximum and minimum of the standard deviation σ and H is the Hurst exponent. In a similar way used to find the correlation dimension, it is possible to approximate a straight line to the logarithmic relationship between R/σ and n. A non-correlated sequence produces a Brownian motion, which holds for $H = 1/2$. Values $H > 1/2$ imply persistence or correlation, i.e., that the trajectory tends to continue its actual direction. Values $H < 1/2$ represent anti-persistence or non-correlation.

7.4 Support Vector Machines (SVM)

Support Vector Machines are a collection of techniques within supervised learning. The objective is to create a limit region between a couple of classes in a multidmensional space [68]. This region or limit margin is defined by a function which, according to an optimizing criterion, ensures the maximum separation between two classes within the feature space.

Given a series of data points to approximate $D = \{(x_1, y_1), ..., (x_n, y_n)\}, x \in \mathbb{R}^N$, where x are the inputs and y are the corresponding outputs in an N-dimensional space, the main objective of the SVM is to find a function $f(x)$ to provide a deviation ε considering the separation of the data of the classes [114]. This function is described in 7.11.

$$f(x) = (w \cdot x) + b; x \in \mathbb{R}^N \tag{7.11}$$

where w is an adjustable step and b is a scalar threshold. In order to find this function, an euclidian norm is considered $||w||^2$ allowing the existence of certain errors between the margins ξ_i and ξ_i^*. The following index is minimized:

$$J = \frac{1}{2}||w||^2 + C\sum_{i=1}^{n}(\xi_i + \xi_i^*) \tag{7.12}$$

subjected to constraints:

$$y_i - (w \cdot x_i + b) \quad \leq \quad \varepsilon + \xi_i \qquad (7.13)$$

$$(w \cdot x_i + b) - y_i \quad \leq \quad \varepsilon + \xi_i^* \qquad (7.14)$$

for $i = 1, 2, ..., n$, $\xi_i, \xi_i^* \geq 0$ and C a variable for allowing the relationship between the slope of the function and the tolerance of the deviation.

SVM are used to classify two linearly separable classes, yet, due to the nature of the data that we are considering, we decided to explore with different kernels with the intention of mapping data to a higher dimension feature space through a nonlinear mapping [208]. Kernels like *Linear, Polynomial, Radial Base Function* and *Sigmoid* were considered, and after several experiments comparing the obtained results [543], the selected kernel was a Radial Base Function (RBF) given by:

$$K(x, x') = \exp\left(-\frac{\gamma(x - x')^2}{\sigma}\right) \qquad (7.15)$$

Since we deal with more than one class, we propose a mutiple SVM model, such that we are able to classify one class vs the others. For this we compare class F vs S and Z, class S vs F and Z, and class Z vs F and S. The results are shown in Section 7.6.

7.5   Embedded classifier

In this section we will describe in detail the classification strategy that we applied, the implementation of the methodology using an All-Programmable System-On-Chip (APSoC) as an embedded system and will give some results.

7.5.1   Model-based design

It has previously been reported that model-based design is a technique used for the design and programming of embedded systems that allows the validation of the correct execution of complex mathematical algorithms, while it allows the software code to be run by the embedded system to be automatically generated by computational tools [329], [523]. In addition, outstanding results with the use of MATLAB and Simulink for the development of embedded systems and mathematical accelerators have already been reported [522]. Based on such reports, C coder, which is a tool that runs over Simulink for the automatic generation of C-language code for some embedded system platforms, has been chosen.

Another paradigm of model-based design with MATLAB and Simulink used in the programming of the classifier is the *embedded function*. An embedded function is a traditional *m* function, which can be incorporated into Simulink as part of a block called state table described with the *StateChart* tool. With *StateChart*, one can control, from the Simulink perspective, the execution order of the *m* code.

7.5.2 Zynq-7000 APSoC

The embedded system chosed for the implementation of the classifier is the Zynq-7000 All-Programmable System-On-Chip, APSoC [296], [567]. This is an FPGA developed by Xilinx and its architecture is shown in Figure 7.2. The APSoC architecture comprises a processing system, a programmable logic section and a set of configurable buses, called *AXI*, for the communication between both sections. The processing system is comprised of a dual-core ARM Cortex-9 embedded processor, which comes equipped with a in-circuit program memory. The programmable logic section is based on architectures such as Artix-7 and Kintex-7 and can be used to add pre-configured peripherals (described in a hardware description language) to the processing system, such as serial communications ports and analog-to-digital converters, to design co-processors. The configuration of the AXI buses depends on the use of the programable logic and its needs of communication with the processing system.

7.5.3 Classifier model

The embedded classifier is composed of each stage of processing shown in Figure 7.3. The mathematical model for the reconstruction of the strange attractor of Section 7.3, as well as the model of Section 7.4, have been described in Simulink along with the parameter configuration necessary for its implementation on the embedded system. It is worth mentioning that, given the necessary interaction between the computer and the embedded system for the information exchange, the embedded system has been configured as *external-mode interface* in Simulink, effectively running as a mathematical accelerator.

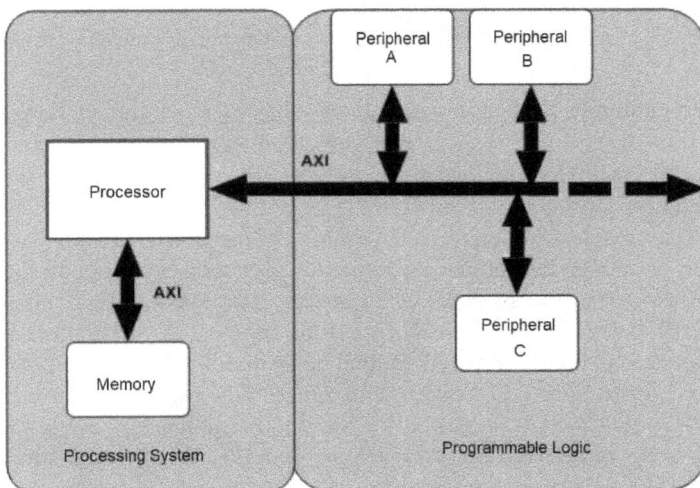

FIGURE 7.2: APSoC architecture.

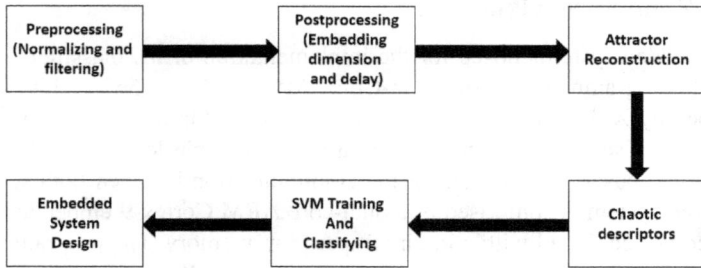

FIGURE 7.3: Components of the embedded classifier.

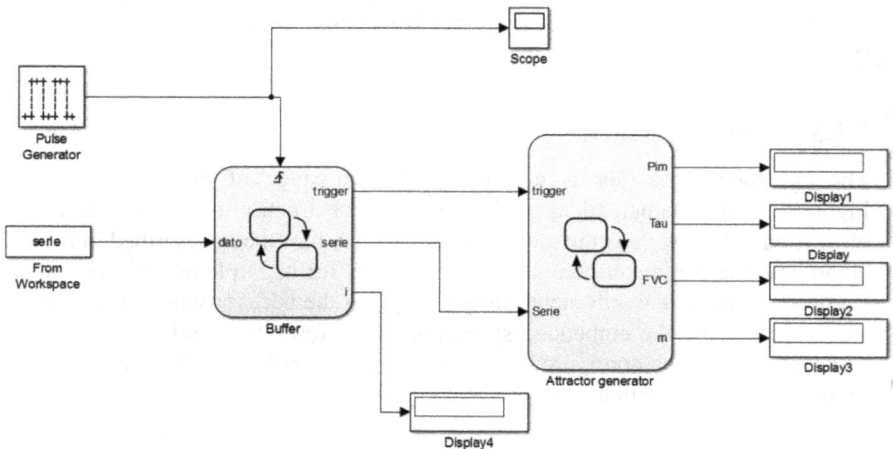

FIGURE 7.4: Reconstruction of the strange attractors.

The Simulink model of Figure 7.4 specifies and executes the algorithm used for the reconstruction of strange attractors. The model comprises two state tables or emphstate charts: *Buffer* and *Atractor generator*. *Buffer* works as a buffer with states that keep storing each sample of the EEG time series until a maximum number of samples is reached, simulating the sampling of the data acquisition system. *Buffer* is also in charge of controlling the processes execution and sending the portion of the time series to process. *Atractor generator* is in charge of calculating the first characteristics for the description of the time series. These characteristics are: average mutual information (AMI), optimal delay coordinates (τ), percentage of false nearest negibours (FNN) and embedding dimension (m). The pulse generator block, *Pulse Generator*, is in charge of stimulating the sampling frequency of the signal. *Atractor generator* includes the models for the generation of the attractors in the form of **MATLAB** embedded functions.

The model for the classification of each signal according to its chaotic descriptors is defined in two stages. The first stage of the model is shown in Figure 7.5. The

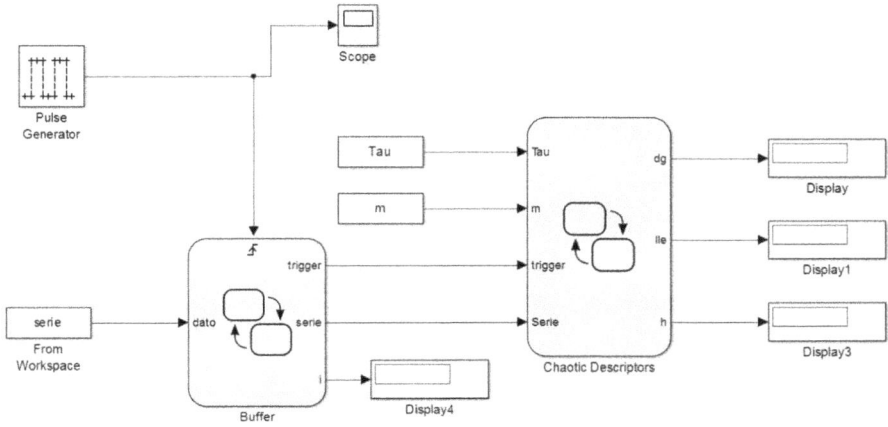

FIGURE 7.5: First stage of the Simulink model for the calculation of the chaotic descriptors.

Buffer block is used for the acquisition of the time series and as a controller of the model through its *trigger* terminal. The emphChaotic descriptors block includes the MATLAB embedded functions for the calculation of the correlation dimension (D_g), the largest Lyapunov exponent (LLE) and the Hurst exponent (H).

The second part of the classifier model involves the use of the SVM models discussed in Section 7.4. The parameters for the RBF Kernel were chosen through heuristic statistics, such as the standard deviation, for the selection of the parameters γ and σ [208].

7.5.4   Strategy of the proposed classification

The resulting classifier model is shown in Figure 7.6, which includes three SVM in one-against-all models. Each SVM has its own Kernal parameter configuration, with the purpose to improve the classification. The *Integrador* is in charge of interpreting the outputs returned by each individual sub-model and providing a general output of the model. The three individual outputs lead to three possible cases to consider:

1. One of the SVM outputs is *true*, while the other two outputs are *false* and the class is correct. Therefore, it is determined that the sample is correctly classified as true positive for the first SVM or true negative for the other two.

2. One of the SVM outputs is *true*, while one of the others or both outputs are *true* and the class is incorrect. Therefore, it is determined that the sample is incorrectly classified as false positive.

3. One of the SVM outputs is *false*, while one of the others or both outputs are *true* and the class is correct. Therefore, it is determined that the sample is incorrectly classified as false negative.

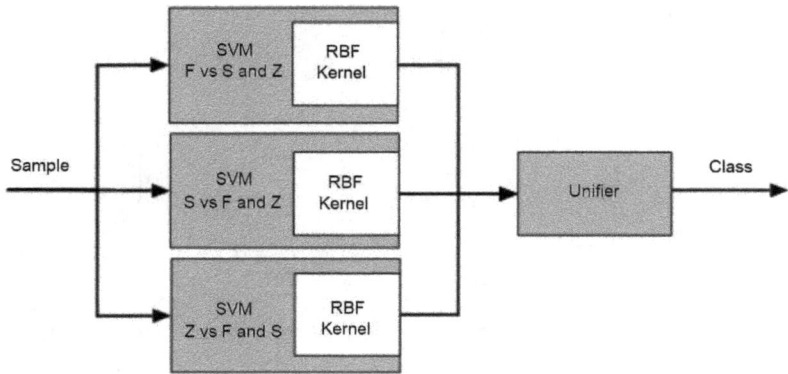

FIGURE 7.6: Classifier model with three SVMs using the RBF Kernel.

In other words, for a sample to be correctly classified it is required that one and only one SVM output is *true*, while the other two outputs are *false* and that the sample effectively belongs to the class it should belong to.

The training of the SVMs is not part of the Simulink model, that is, the variables that resulted from the off-line training have been provided to the classifier model in the form of static variables or vectors in memory for each SVM. The retraining of the SVMs require the updated variables to be added again to the Simulink environment. The models of the SVMs consist of MATLAB embedded functions, one function for each, which execute sequentially in response to the occurrence of the *trigger* signal, provided by the *Buffer* block shown in Figure 7.5. The parameters used by the RBF Kernel are $\gamma/\delta = 0.2$ for F vs S and Z, $\gamma/\delta = 0.5$ for S vs F and Z and $\gamma/\delta = 0.15$ for Z vs F and S.

7.6 Case study

In this section, results for the application of the proposed strategy are shown. We consider the Bonn epilepsy database [27] and show classifications for healthy and epilepsy-diagnosed subjects, free of seizure and during a seizure.

7.6.1 Preprocessing

During the acquisiton of the EEG signals, noise or undesirable frequencies are added in the brain frequency bands, thus it is needed to filter those signals. Although the signals within the used database were already filtered, another band-pass FIR filter was applied with a range of frequencies of 0.53–85 Hz. The time series were normalized using the scaled value method to obtain values between 0 and 1. The purpose was to facilitate the computational analysis by avoiding negative numbers and statistical bias.

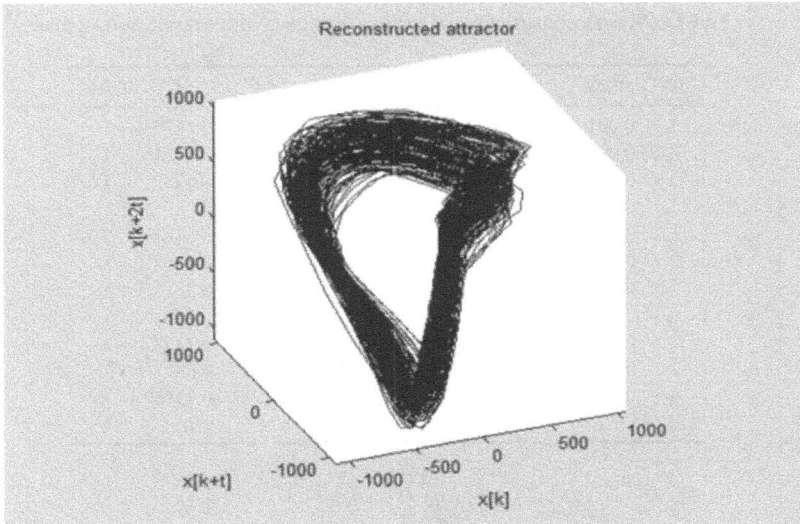

FIGURE 7.7: Three dimension projection of the reconstruction of the attractor of a sample of the S set with $m = 6$ and $\tau = 3$.

The last stage of classifier preprocessing is the reconstruction of the strange attractors of each of the EEG time series. Figure 7.7 shows a projection of an attractor in three dimensions for $m = 6$ and $\tau = 3$ with $R_{TOL} = 15$ and $A_{TOL} = 2$. In a visual way, it is possible to note a certain quasi-periodical pattern.

7.6.2   Postprocessing

Due to the computational complexity of certain algorithms, such as the computation of the Euclidean distances between all the points of the attractor, it was deemed necessary to do a windowing of the signal and analyzing sections of it to reduce the processing effort of the Simulink models. The tests were conducted with windows of 32, 64 and 128 samples of the signal. The 64-sample window was finally chosen because it carries the signal information necessary for its characterization with which to proceed with the training of the classifier.

7.6.3   Processing results

Table 7.1 shows the values of PIM, (τ), FVC, m, (D_g), LLE and (H) of the F, S and Z sets. D_g, LLE and H are used as chaotic descriptors for the training of the classifier. Figure 7.8 shows these values in the descriptors space.

TABLE 7.1: Reconstruction of strange attractors and chaotic descriptors.

ID	PIM	τ	%FVC	m	D_g	LLE	H	Class
1	0.0019	4	0.0000	13	4.96	0.3142	0.7420	F
2	0.0000	14	0.0279	14	3.38	0.0760	0.7734	F
3	0.0020	2	0.0270	6	2.92	0.3309	0.6957	F
...	...	...	...	...	...	...	...	...
1	0.0017	1	0.0000	6	2.38	0.0297	0.5377	S
2	0.0020	1	0.0000	6	2.37	0.1709	0.6014	S
3	0.0014	3	8.3045	8	3.42	0.1696	0.5116	S
...	...	...	...	...	...	...	...	...
1	0.0018	5	0.0261	14	1.37	0.3321	0.7257	Z
2	0.0022	1	0.0000	5	1.05	0.0392	0.6897	Z
3	0.0015	1	0.0000	6	1.21	0.0225	0.7378	Z
...	...	...	...	...	...	...	...	...

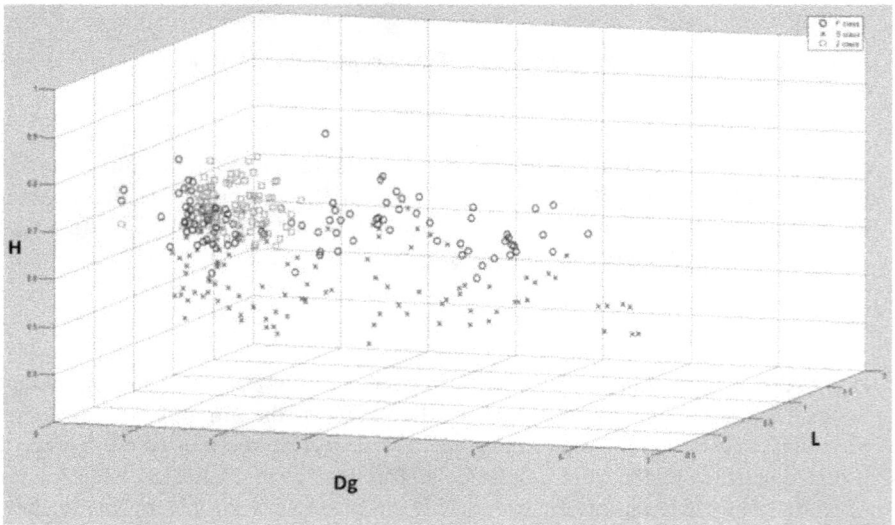

FIGURE 7.8: Values in the descriptors space according to class: F (circles), S (crosses) y Z (squares).

7.6.4 Classification results

Table 7.2 shows the results obtained from the SVMs with the parameters described above (γ/σ), the RBF Kernel and a direct training, that is, with all the samples validated with the same trained ones.

TABLE 7.2: Classification results with the SVMs.

SVM	No. of support vectors	b	correct	accuracy (%)
F vs S y Z	238	-0.3382	293	97.67
S vs F y Z	96	-0.3973	296	98.67
Z vs F y S	269	0.6205	296	98.67
General			286	95.33

7.7 Discussion

This work reports the results obtained from different time-series analysis techniques of EEG signals of healthy patients and patients diagnosed with epilepsy, including dynamic systems theory and chaotic descriptors and diverse pattern classification tools used in Artificial Intelligence techniques. Such techniques and tools were implemented on an embedded system.

With the public database from the Center of Epileptology of the University of Bonn, the percentage of correctly classified samples was 95.33, using direct training with a classifier based on three Support Vector Machines and such chaotic descriptors as correlation dimension, largest Lyapunov exponent and Hurst exponent.

The chosen embedded system was APSoC Zynq-7000 from Xilinx, which comprises a processing system section based on dual-core ARM Cortex-9 and a programmable logic section. For this work, MATLAB C Coder was used, which automatically generates C-language code from the *StateChart* and Simulink tools. The generated code is executed by the processing system of the APSoC. The resulting embedded system is programmed with the chaotic descriptors and the classifier and executes them from a mathematical accelerator paradigm. However, not all the SVM processing is run by the embedded system. The training is run off-line and the parameters resulting from the training are then programmed in the embedded system to proceed with the classification.

It is worth noticing the relevance of the study of epilepsy with encephalogram signals in developing countries, since statistically their population is most affected by this disease. The authors deem necessary that tests with a more clinical approach and different public databases of EEG signals (with different patients and different clinical cases) be conducted. This would lead to an embedded system with a higher diversification of data and a more robust training.

Bibliography

[1] Sithara A, Abraham Thomas and Dominic Mathew. Study of mfcc and ihc feature extraction methods with probabilistic acoustic models for speaker biometric applications. *Procedia Computer Science*, 143: 267–276, 2018. 8th International Conference on Advances in Computing and Communications (ICACC-2018).

[2] AH Aswathy, GM Sukumar, MS Swapnil, VA Kumar, A Krishna et al. Solar powered intelligent electric wheel chair with health monitoring system. In *2017 International Conference on Technological Advancements in Power and Energy (TAP Energy)*, pp. 1–5, December 2017. Journal Abbreviation: 2017 International Conference on Technological Advancements in Power and Energy (TAP Energy).

[3] Henry DI Abarbanel and Matthew B Kennel. Local false nearest neighbors and dynamical dimensions from observed chaotic data. *Physical Review E*, 47(5): 3057, 1993.

[4] Bardia Abbasi and Daniel M Goldenholz. Machine learning applications in epilepsy. *Epilepsia*, 60(10): 2037–2047, 2019.

[5] Nicholas S Abend, Frances E Jensen, Terrie E Inder and Joseph J Volpe. Neonatal seizures. In *Volpe's Neurology of the Newborn*, pp. 275–321. Elsevier, 2018.

[6] Khalid Abualsaud, Massudi Mahmuddin, Mohammad Saleh and Amr Mohamed. Ensemble classifier for epileptic seizure detection for imperfect eeg data. *The Scientific World Journal*, 2015, 2015.

[7] Evrim Acar, Canan A Bingol, Haluk Bingol and Bülent Yener. Computational analysis of epileptic focus localization. In *Proc. of the Fourth IASTED International Conference on Biomedical Engineering*, p. 317, 2006.

[8] Gizem Acar, Ozberk Ozturk, Ata Jedari Golparvar, Tamador Alkhidir Elboshra, Karl Böhringer et al. Wearable and flexible textile electrodes for biopotential signal monitoring: A review. *Electronics*, 8(5): 479, April 2019.

[9] S Ackerman. Major structures and functions of the brain. *Discovering the Brain*, 1992.

[10] Milan Adámek, Miroslav Matỳsek and Petr Neumann. Security of biometric systems. *Procedia Engineering*, 100: 169–176, 2015.

[11] Md Nasim Adnan, Md Zahidul Islam et al. Forex++: A new framework for knowledge discovery from decision forests. *Australasian Journal of Information Systems*, 21, 2017.

[12] Hamid K Aghajan, Juan Carlos Augusto and Ramón López-Cózar Delgado. *Human-centric Interfaces for Ambient Intelligence*. Academic Press, 2009.

[13] David W Aha, Dennis Kibler and Marc K Albert. Instance-based learning algorithms. *Machine Learning*, 6(1): 37–66, 1991.

[14] Ahmed Awad E Ahmed and Issa Traore. A new biometric technology based on mouse dynamics. *IEEE Transactions on Dependable and Secure Computing*, 4(3): 165–179, 2007.

[15] Qingsong Ai, Anqi Chen, Kun Chen, Quan Liu, Tichao Zhou et al. Feature extraction of four-class motor imagery eeg signals based on functional brain network. *Journal of Neural Engineering*, 16(2): 026032, 2019.

[16] Zahid Akhtar, Abdenour Hadid, Mark Nixon, Massimo Tistarelli, Jean-Luc Dugelay et al. Biometrics: In search of identity and security *(q & a)*. *IEEE MultiMedia*, pp. 1–1: 10, 2018.

[17] Neamah Al-Naffakh, Nathan Clarke, Paul Dowland and Fudong Li. Activity recognition using wearable computing. In *2016 11th International Conference for Internet Technology and Secured Transactions (ICITST)*, pp. 189–195. IEEE, 2016.

[18] Mashael Aldayel, Mourad Ykhlef and Abeer Al-Nafjan. Deep learning for eeg-based preference classification in neuromarketing. *Applied Sciences*, 10(4), 2020.

[19] Abdullah A Aljumah, Mohammad Khubeb Siddiqui and Mohammad Gulam Ahamad. Application of classification based data mining technique in diabetes care. *Journal of Applied Sciences*, 416–422, 2013.

[20] Lujambio I Alonso, SF Arturo, Nava B Lucero, Piña W Cesar, Escobar Z Maria Teresa et al. Discapacidad motriz: Guía didáctica para la inclusión en educación inicial y básica. *Cons Nac Fom Educ*, 2010.

[21] Gaseb Alotibi, Nathan Clarke, Fudong Li and Steven Furnell. User profiling from network traffic via novel application-level interactions. In *Internet Technology and Secured Transactions (ICITST), 2016 11th International Conference for*, pp. 279–285. IEEE, 2016.

[22] Ethem Alpaydin. *Introduction to Machine Learning*. MIT Press, 2020.

[23] Abdulaziz Alzubaidi and Jugal Kalita. Authentication of smartphone users using behavioral biometrics. *IEEE Communications Surveys & Tutorials*, 18(3): 1998–2026, 2016.

[24] Abdulaziz Alzubaidi and Jugal Kalita. Authentication of smartphone users using behavioral biometrics. *IEEE Communications Surveys Tutorials*, 18(3): 1998–2026, thirdquarter, 2016.

[25] John R Anderson, Shawn Betts, Jennifer L Ferris and Jon M Fincham. Neural imaging to track mental states while using an intelligent tutoring system. *Proceedings of the National Academy of Sciences*, 107(15): 7018–7023, 2010.

[26] Ralph G Andrzejak, Klaus Lehnertz, Florian Mormann, Christoph Rieke, Peter David et al. Indications of nonlinear deterministic and finite-dimensional structures in time series of brain electrical activity: Dependence on recording region and brain state. *Physical Review E*, 64(6): 061907, 2001.

[27] Ralph G Andrzejak, Klaus Lehnertz, Florian Mormann, Christoph Rieke, Peter David et al. Indications of nonlinear deterministic and finite-dimensional structures in time series of brain electrical activity: Dependence on recording region and brain state. *Physical Review E*, 64(6): 061907, 2001.

[28] Scott Anjewierden, Jeffrey Humpherys, Martin J LaPage, S Yukiko Asaki and Peter F Aziz. Detection of tachyarrhythmias in a large cohort of infants using direct-to-consumer heart rate monitoring. *The Journal of Pediatrics*, 232: 147–153.e1, 2021.

[29] Leonidas Anthopoulos. Smart utopia VS smart reality: Learning by experience from 10 smart city cases. *Cities*, 63: 128–148, 2017.

[30] Milos Antonijevic, Miodrag Zivkovic, Sladjana Arsic and Aleksandar Jevremovic. Using ai-based classification techniques to process eeg data collected during the visual short-term memory assessment. *Journal of Sensors*, 2020, 2020.

[31] Anett Antony and R Gopikakumari. Speaker identification based on combination of mfcc and umrt based features. *Procedia Computer Science*, 143: 250–257, 2018. 8th International Conference on Advances in Computing and Communications (ICACC-2018).

[32] Maxwell Fordjour Antwi-Afari, Heng Li, Yantao Yu and Liulin Kong. Wearable insole pressure system for automated detection and classification of awkward working postures in construction workers. *Automation in Construction*, 96: 433–441, 2018.

[33] Diego E Arias, Esteban J Pino, Pablo Aqueveque and Dorothy W Curtis. Unobtrusive support system for prevention of dangerous health conditions in wheelchair users. *Mobile Information Systems*, 2016: 4568241, July 2016. Publisher: Hindawi Publishing Corporation.

[34] Jason F Arnold and Robert M Sade. Wearable technologies in collegiate sports: The ethics of collecting biometric data from student-athletes. *The American Journal of Bioethics: AJOB*, 17(1): 67–70, Jan 2017.

[35] Christopher Arthmann and I-Ping Li. Neuromarketing-the art and science of marketing and neurosciences enabled by iot technologies. *IIC Journal of Innovation*, 1–10, 2017.

[36] Jessica Askamp and Michel JAM van Putten. Mobile eeg in epilepsy. *International Journal of Psychophysiology*, 91(1): 30–35, 2014.

[37] Musbah Abdulkarim Musbah Ataya and Musab AM Ali. Acceptance of website security on e-banking. A-review. In *2019 IEEE 10th Control and System Graduate Research Colloquium (ICSGRC)*, pp. 201–206, 2019.

[38] Emrah Aydemir, Turker Tuncer, Sengul Dogan and Musa Unsal. A novel biometric recognition method based on multi kernelled bijection octal pattern using gait sound. *Applied Acoustics*, 173: 107701, 2021.

[39] Hyun Jae Baek, Gih Sung Chung, Ko Keun Kim and Kwang Suk Park. A smart health monitoring chair for nonintrusive measurement of biological signals. *IEEE Transactions on Information Technology in Biomedicine: A Publication of the IEEE Engineering in Medicine and Biology Society*, 16(1): 150–158, January 2012. Place: United States.

[40] Yang Bai, Xiaoli Li and Zhenhu Liang. Nonlinear neural dynamics. In *EEG Signal Processing and Feature Extraction*, pp. 215–240. Springer, 2019.

[41] Sylvain Baillet, Karl Friston and Robert Oostenveld. Academic software applications for electromagnetic brain mapping using meg and eeg, 2011.

[42] Samer Ahmed Bakr. Digital jewellery and machine learning methods for analysing player performance in sports. *Annals of the Romanian Society for Cell Biology*, 25(6): 2093–2103, 2021.

[43] Asok Bandyopadhyay and Basabi Chakraborty. Development of online handwriting recognition system: A case study with handwritten bangla character. In *Nature & Biologically Inspired Computing, 2009. NaBIC 2009. World Congress on*, pp. 514–519. IEEE, 2009.

[44] R Barea, L Boquete, M Mazo and E López. Wheelchair guidance strategies using EOG. *Journal of Intelligent and Robotic Systems*, 34(3): 279–299, July 2002.

[45] Silvio Barra, Aniello Castiglione, Maria De Marsico, Michele Nappi and Kim Kwang Raymond Choo. Cloud-based biometrics (biometrics as a service) for smart cities, nations, and beyond. *IEEE Cloud Computing*, 5(5): 92–100, 2018.

[46] Silvio Barra, Aniello Castiglione, Maria De Marsico, Michele Nappi and Kim-Kwang Raymond Choo. Cloud-based biometrics (biometrics as a service) for smart cities, nations, and beyond. *IEEE Cloud Computing*, 5(5): 92–100, 2018.

[47] Silvio Barra, Kim-Kwang Raymond Choo, Michele Nappi, Arcangelo Castiglione, Fabio Narducci et al. Biometrics-as-a-service: Cloud-based technology, systems, and applications. *IEEE Cloud Computing*, 5(4): 33–37, 2018.

[48] Barbara Rita Barricelli, Elena Casiraghi, Jessica Gliozzo, Alessandro Petrini and Stefano Valtolina. Human digital twin for fitness management. *IEEE Access*, 8: 26637–26664, 2020.

[49] Mary Bates. The rise of biometrics in sports. *IEEE Pulse*, 11(3): 25–28, 2020.

[50] Anthony D Bateson, Heidi A Baseler, Kevin S Paulson, Fayyaz Ahmed and Aziz UR Asghar. Categorisation of mobile eeg: A researcher's perspective. *BioMed Research International*, 2017, 2017.

[51] A Benard, EC Bos-Levenbach et al. Het uitzetten van waarnemingen op waarschijnlijkheids-papier1. *Statistica Neerlandica*, 7(3): 163–173, 1953.

[52] Clara Benevolo, Renata Paola Dameri and Beatrice D Auria. Smart mobility in smart city. *Empowering Organizations: Enabling Platforms and Artefacts*, 11: 315, 2016.

[53] Hans Berger. Über das elektroenkephalogramm des menschen. *Archiv für psychiatrie und nervenkrankheiten*, 87(1): 527–570, 1929.

[54] Rebecca A Bernert, David A Luckenbaugh, Wallace C Duncan, Naomi G Iwata, Elizabeth D Ballard et al. Sleep architecture parameters as a putative biomarker of suicidal ideation in treatment-resistant depression. *Journal of Affective Disorders*, 208: 309–315, 2017.

[55] Tim Betts. Epilepsy, psychiatry and learning difficulty. *Seizure-European Journal of Epilepsy*, 7(5): 431, 1998.

[56] Eckhard Beubler. *Compendium of Pharmacology: Common Drugs in Practice*. Springer-Verlag, 2017.

[57] Renu Bhatia. Biometrics and face recognition techniques. *International Journal of Advanced Research in Computer Science and Software Engineering*, 3(5), 2013.

[58] Mrinal Kanti Bhowmik, Priya Saha, Anu Singha, Debotosh Bhattacharjee and Paramartha Dutta. Enhancement of robustness of face recognition system through reduced gaussianity in log-ica. *Expert Systems with Applications*, 116: 96–107, 2019.

[59] Nima Bigdely-Shamlo, Tim Mullen, Christian Kothe, Kyung-Min Su and Kay A Robbins. The prep pipeline: Standardized preprocessing for large-scale eeg analysis. *Frontiers in Neuroinformatics*, 9: 16, 2015.

[60] Javad Birjandtalab, Vipul Nataraj Jarmale, Mehrdad Nourani and Jay Harvey. Imbalance learning using neural networks for seizure detection. In *2018 IEEE Biomedical Circuits and Systems Conference (BioCAS)*, pp. 1–4. IEEE, 2018.

[61] Javad Birjandtalab, Maziyar Baran Pouyan and Mehrdad Nourani. Unsupervised eeg analysis for automated epileptic seizure detection. In *First International Workshop on Pattern Recognition*, volume 10011, p. 100110M. International Society for Optics and Photonics, 2016.

[62] Warren T Blume, Hans O Lüders, Eli Mizrahi, Carlo Tassinari, Walter van Emde Boas et al. Glossary of descriptive terminology for ictal semiology: Report of the ilae task force on classification and terminology. *Epilepsia*, 42(9): 1212–1218, 2001.

[63] Addo Boafo, Roseanne Armitage, Stephanie Greenham, Paniz Tavakoli, Alyson Dale et al. Sleep architecture in adolescents hospitalized during a suicidal crisis. *Sleep Medicine*, 56: 41–46, 2019.

[64] M Bolanos, H Nazeran and E Haltiwanger. Comparison of heart rate variability signal features derived from electrocardiography and photoplethysmography in healthy individuals. In *2006 International Conference of the IEEE Engineering in Medicine and Biology Society*, pp. 4289–4294. IEEE, 2006.

[65] Bonneau Vincent, Probot Laurent and Lefebvre Virginie. Biometrics technologies: A key enabler for future digital services. Digital Transformation Monitor, European Commission. Available at https://ati. ec.europa.eu/sites/default/files/2020-07/Biometrics%20technologies%20 -%20a%20key%20enabler%20for%20future%20digital%20services%20 %28v2%29.pdf (accessed: 2021-05-11), 2018.

[66] Nikolaos V Boulgouris, Dimitrios Hatzinakos and Konstantinos N Plataniotis. Gait recognition: A challenging signal processing technology for biometric identification. *IEEE Signal Processing Magazine*, 22(6): 78–90, 2005.

[67] Patrick Bours and Adrian Evensen. The shakespeare experiment: Preliminary results for the recognition of a person based on the sound of walking. In *Security Technology (ICCST), 2017 International Carnahan Conference on*, pp. 1–6. IEEE, 2017.

[68] Brandon H Boyle. *Support Vector Machines: Data Analysis, Machine Learning and Applications*. Nova Science Publ., 2011.

[69] Hakan Boz, Aytuğ Arslan and Erdoğan Koc. Neuromarketing aspect of tourism pricing psychology. *Tourism Management Perspectives*, 23: 119–128, 2017.

[70] Simón Brailowsky. *Epilepsia: Enfermedad sagrada del cerebro*. Secretaría de Educación Pública., 1999.

[71] Trevor Braun, Benjamin CM Fung, Farkhund Iqbal and Babar Shah. Security and privacy challenges in smart cities. *Sustainable Cities and Society*, 39(August 2017): 499–507, 2018.

[72] Keith W Brawner and Avelino J Gonzalez. Modelling a learner's affective state in real time to improve intelligent tutoring effectiveness. *Theoretical Issues in Ergonomics Science*, 17(2): 183–210, 2016.

[73] Leo Breiman. Bagging predictors. *Machine Learning*, 24(2): 123–140, 1996.

[74] Pam Briggs and Patric Olivier. Biometrie daemons: Authentication via electronic pets. *Conference on Human Factors in Computing Systems—Proceedings*, 1(January): 2423–2431, 2008.

[75] Koen Bruynseels, Filippo Santoni de Sio and Jeroen van den Hoven. Digital twins in health care: Ethical implications of an emerging engineering paradigm. *Frontiers in Genetics*, 9(Feb): 1–11, 2018.

[76] Attaullah Buriro, Sandeep Gupta and Bruno Crispo. Evaluation of motion-based touch-typing biometrics for online banking. In *2017 International Conference of the Biometrics Special Interest Group (BIOSIG)*, pp. 1–5, 2017.

[77] Adrian Burns, Barry R Greene, Michael J McGrath, Terrance J O'Shea, Benjamin Kuris et al. Shimmer™–a wireless sensor platform for noninvasive biomedical research. *IEEE Sensors Journal*, 10(9): 1527–1534, 2010.

[78] Christoph Busch. Facing the future of biometrics. Demand for safety and security in the public and private sectors is driving research in this rapidly growing field. *EMBO Reports*, 7 Spec No(Spec No): S23–5, Jul 2006.

[79] C. Yang, G. Cheung and V. Stankovic. Estimating heart rate and rhythm via 3D motion tracking in depth video. *IEEE Transactions on Multimedia*, 19(7): 1625–1636, July 2017.

[80] Yiyu Cai, Wouter van Joolingen and Zachary Walker, editors. VR, *Simulations and Serious Games for Education*. Gaming Media and Social Effects. Springer Singapore, Singapore, 2019.

[81] Z Cao, E Koukharenko, RN Torah, J Tudor and SP Beeby. Flexible screen printed thick film thermoelectric generator with reduced material resistivity. *Journal of Physics: Conference Series*, 557: 012016, Nov 2014.

[82] Raffaele Cappelli, Matteo Ferrara and Davide Maltoni. Minutia cylindercode: A new representation and matching technique for fingerprint recognition. *IEEE Transactions on Pattern Analysis and Machine Intelligence*, 32(12): 2128–2141, 2010.

[83] A Casiano and H González. Automatic classification of eeg epileptic patterns using chaotic descriptors. In *Congreso Nacional de Control Automático*, 2005.

[84] Alexander J Casson. Wearable eeg and beyond. *Biomedical Engineering Letters*, 9(1): 53–71, 2019.

[85] Alexander J Casson, Shelagh Smith, John S Duncan and Esther Rodriguez-Villegas. Wearable eeg: what is it, why is it needed and what does it entail? In *2008 30th Annual International Conference of the IEEE Engineering in Medicine and Biology Society*, pp. 5867–5870. IEEE, 2008.

[86] Denisse Castaneda, Aibhlin Esparza, Mohammad Ghamari, Cinna Soltanpur and Homer Nazeran. A review on wearable photoplethysmography sensors and their potential future applications in health care. *International Journal of Biosensors & Bioelectronics*, 4(4): 195, 2018.

[87] David R Causton, Jill C Venus et al. *The Biometry of Plant Growth*. Edward Arnold., 1981.

[88] Elena Ceseracciu, Zimi Sawacha, Silvia Fantozzi, Matteo Cortesi, Giorgio Gatta et al. Markerless analysis of front crawl swimming. *Journal of Biomechanics*, 44(12): 2236–2242, 2011.

[89] Harish Chander, Reuben F Burch, Purva Talegaonkar, David Saucier, Tony Luczak et al. Wearable stretch sensors for human movement monitoring and fall detection in ergonomics. *International Journal of Environmental Research and Public Health*, 17(10), May 2020.

[90] Won-Du Chang. Electrooculograms for human-computer interaction: A review. *Sensors (Basel, Switzerland)*, 19(12), June 2019.

[91] Jack Chaplin, Giovanna Martinez-Arellano and Andrea Mazzoleni. Digital twins and intelligent decision making. In *Digital Manufacturing for SMEs*. Digital Manufacturing Training, 2020.

[92] Nitesh V Chawla, Kevin W Bowyer, Lawrence O Hall and W Philip Kegelmeyer. Smote: synthetic minority over-sampling technique. *Journal of Artificial Intelligence Research*, 16: 321–357, 2002.

[93] Duo Chen, Suiren Wan, Jing Xiang and Forrest Sheng Bao. A high-performance seizure detection algorithm based on discrete wavelet transform (dwt) and eeg. *PloS One*, 12(3): e0173138, 2017.

[94] Hai Chen and Mohamad Z Koubeissi. Electroencephalography in epilepsy evaluation. *Continuum: Lifelong Learning in Neurology*, 25(2): 431–453, 2019.

[95] Qingguo Chen and Liqin Tang. A wearable blood oxygen saturation monitoring system based on bluetooth low energy technology. *Computer Communications*, 160: 101–110, 2020.

[96] Xin Chen, Haixia Liu, Yile Wu, Kun Xuan, Tianming Zhao et al. Characteristics of sleep architecture in autism spectrum disorders: A meta-analysis based on polysomnographic research. *Psychiatry Research*, 296: 113677, 2021.

[97] Eric-Juwei Cheng, Kuang-Pen Chou, Shantanu Rajora, Bo-Hao Jin, M Tanveer et al. Deep sparse representation classifier for facial recognition and detection system. *Pattern Recognition Letters*, 125: 71–77, 2019.

[98] Ohbet Cheon, George Naufal and Bita A Kash. When workplace wellness programs work: Lessons learned from a large employer in texas. *American Journal of Health Education*, 51(1): 31–39, 2020.

[99] Cheng-Yi Chiang, Nai-Fu Chang, Tung-Chien Chen, Hong-Hui Chen and Liang-Gee Chen. Seizure prediction based on classification of eeg synchronization patterns with on-line retraining and post-processing scheme. In *2011 Annual International Conference of the IEEE Engineering in Medicine and Biology Society*, pp. 7564–7569. IEEE, 2011.

[100] Sang Han Choi, Minho Lee, Yijun Wang and Bo Hong. Estimation of optimal location of eeg reference electrode for motor imagery based bci using fmri. In *2006 International Conference of the IEEE Engineering in Medicine and Biology Society*, pp. 1193–1196. IEEE, 2006.

[101] Ki H Chon, Christopher G Scully and Sheng Lu. Approximate entropy for all signals. *IEEE Engineering in Medicine and Biology Magazine*, 28(6): 18–23, 2009.

[102] Hsi-Chiang Chou, Yi-Ming Wang and Huai-Yuan Chang. Design intelligent wheelchair with ECG measurement and wireless transmission function. *Technology and Health Care: Official Journal of the European Society for Engineering and Medicine*, 24 Suppl 1: S345–355, 2015. Place: Netherlands.

[103] Yu-kai Chou. *Actionable Gamification Beyond Points, Badges, and Leaderboards.* CreateSpace Independent Publishing Platform, 2015.

[104] Michael X Cohen. Where does eeg come from and what does it mean? *Trends in Neurosciences*, 40(4): 208–218, 2017.

[105] Mike X Cohen. *Analyzing Neural Time Series Data: Theory and Practice.* MIT Press, 2014.

[106] Tommaso Colombo, Giulio Panzani, Sergio M Savaresi and Pascal Paparo. Absolute driving style estimation for ground vehicles. In *Control*

Technology and Applications (CCTA), 2017 IEEE Conference on,
pp. 2196–2201. IEEE, 2017.

[107] Patrick Connor and Arun Ross. Biometric recognition by gait: A survey of modalities and features. *Computer Vision and Image Understanding,* 167: 1–27, 2018.

[108] Nicholas R Cooper, Ignazio Puzzo, Adam D Pawley, Ruby A Bowes-Mulligan, Emma V Kirkpatrick et al. Bridging a yawning chasm: Eeg investigations into the debate concerning the role of the human mirror neuron system in contagious yawning. *Cognitive, Affective, & Behavioral Neuroscience,* 12(2): 393–405, 2012.

[109] Patricia M Corby, Titus Schleyer, Heiko Spallek, Thomas C Hart, Robert J Weyant et al. Using biometrics for participant identification in a research study: A case report. *Journal of the American Medical Informatics Association: JAMIA,* 13(2): 233–235, 2006.

[110] Corinna Cortes and Vladimir Vapnik. Support-vector networks. *Machine Learning,* 20(3): 273–297, 1995.

[111] Madalena Costa, Ary L Goldberger and C-K Peng. Multiscale entropy analysis of complex physiologic time series. *Physical Review Letters,* 89(6): 068102, 2002.

[112] L Coutier, P Bierme, M Thieux, A Guyon, I Ioan et al. The role of sleep laboratory polygraphy in the evaluation of obstructive sleep apnea syndrome in robin infants. *Sleep Medicine,* 72: 59–64, 2020.

[113] Coronavirus COVID-19 (2019-nCoV). Available at https://gisanddata. maps.arcgis.com/apps/opsdashboard/index.html (accessed: 2020-10-20).

[114] Nello Cristianini, John Shawe-Taylor et al. *An Introduction to Support Vector Machines and other Kernel-based Learning Methods.* Cambridge University Press, 2000.

[115] Nicholas Cummins, Alice Baird and Björn W Schuller. Speech analysis for health: Current state-of-the-art and the increasing impact of deep learning. *Methods,* 151: 41–54, 2018. Health Informatics and Translational Data Analytics.

[116] Emily E Cust, Alice J Sweeting, Kevin Ball and Sam Robertson. Machine and deep learning for sport-specific movement recognition: A systematic review of model development and performance. *Journal of Sports Sciences,* 37(5): 568–600, Mar 2019.

[117] Ryan Cvelbar. "A fitbit for your brain"-elon musk, sci-fi or attainable? *Osmosis Magazine*, 2020(2): 9, 2020.

[118] D Krzesimowski and Z Ciota. Voice signal processing for patiens with stroke hospitalisation. In *2009 MIXDES-16th International Conference Mixed Design of Integrated Circuits & Systems*, pp. 693–696, June 2009. Journal Abbreviation: 2009 MIXDES-16th International Conference Mixed Design of Integrated Circuits & Systems.

[119] Harihara Dadi and PG Mohan. Improved face recognition rate using hog features and svm classifier. *IOSR Journal of Electronics and Communication Engineering (IOSR-JECE)*, 11: 34–44, 04 2016.

[120] Georgios Dafoulas, Jerome Samuels-Clarke, Cristiano Cardoso Maia, Almaas A. Ali and Ariadni Tsiakara. Offering smarter learning support through the use of biometrics. In *2019 26th International Conference on Telecommunications (ICT)*, pp. 270–274, 2019.

[121] Georgios A Dafoulas, C Maia, JS Clarke, A Ali and J Augusto. Investigating the role of biometrics in education—the use of sensor data in collaborative learning. *International Association for Development of the Information Society*, pp. 115–123, 2018.

[122] Georgios A Dafoulas, Cristiano Cardoso Maia, Jerome Samuels Clarke, Almaas Ali and Juan Augusto. Investigating the role of biometrics in education—The use of sensor data in collaborative learning. *MCCSIS 2018—Multi Conference on Computer Science and Information Systems; Proceedings of the International Conferences on e-Learning 2018*, 2018-July: 115–123, 2018.

[123] Massimiliano de Zambotti, Aimee Goldstone, Stephanie Claudatos, Ian M Colrain and Fiona C Baker. A validation study of fitbit charge 2™ compared with polysomnography in adults. *Chronobiology International*, 35(4): 465–476, 2018. PMID: 29235907.

[124] Steven F DeFroda, Charles A Thigpen and Peter K Kriz. Two-dimensional video analysis of youth and adolescent pitching biomechanics: A tool for the common athlete. *Current Sports Medicine Reports*, 15(5): 350–358, 2016.

[125] Guillermo Del Castillo, Steven Skaar, Antonio Cardenas and Linda Fehr. A sonar approach to obstacle detection for a vision-based autonomous wheelchair. *Robotics and Autonomous Systems*, 54(12): 967–981, December 2006.

[126] K Delac and M Grgic. A survey of biometric recognition methods. In *Proceedings. Elmar-2004. 46th International Symposium on Electronics in Marine*, pp. 184–193, 2004.

[127] Norman Delanty, Carl J Vaughan and Jacqueline A French. Medical causes of seizures. *The Lancet*, 352(9125): 383–390, 1998.

[128] Parwinder Kaur Dhillon and Sheetal Kalra. A lightweight biometrics based remote user authentication scheme for iot services. *Journal of Information Security and Applications*, 34: 255–270, 2017.

[129] Abigail Dickinson, Charlotte DiStefano, Damla Senturk and Shafali Spurling Jeste. Peak alpha frequency is a neural marker of cognitive function across the autism spectrum. *European Journal of Neuroscience*, 47(6): 643–651, 2018.

[130] James P Dieffenderfer, Henry Goodell, Brinnae Bent, Eric Beppler, Rochana Jayakumar et al. Wearable wireless sensors for chronic respiratory disease monitoring. In *2015 IEEE 12th International Conference onWearable and Implantable Body Sensor Networks (BSN)*, pp. 1–6, 2015.

[131] Ridha Djemal, Khalil AlSharabi, Sutrisno Ibrahim and Abdullah Alsuwailem. Eeg-based computer aided diagnosis of autism spectrum disorder using wavelet, entropy, and ann. *BioMed Research International*, 2017, 2017.

[132] Sidney D'Mello, Ed Dieterle and Angela Duckworth. Advanced, analytic, automated (aaa) measurement of engagement during learning. *Educational Psychologist*, 52(2): 104–123, 2017.

[133] Sidney D'Mello, Andrew Olney, Claire Williams and Patrick Hays. Gaze tutor: A gaze-reactive intelligent tutoring system. *International Journal of Human-Computer Studies*, 70(5): 377–398, 2012.

[134] TW Do. *Ambulatory EEG (Illustrated Ed.)*. Demos Medical Publishing, 2017.

[135] C Doege, R Kleiss, U Stephani and S von Spiczak. Myoclonic-astatic epilepsy. *Magazine f "ur Epileptology*, 27(2): 105–111, 2014.

[136] Corinna Doege, Theodor W May, Michael Siniatchkin, Sarah von Spiczak, Ulrich Stephani et al. Myoclonic astatic epilepsy (doose syndrome)–a lamotrigine responsive epilepsy? *European Journal of Paediatric Neurology*, 17(1): 29–35, 2013.

[137] Cristian Donos, Matthias Dümpelmann and Andreas Schulze-Bonhage. Early seizure detection algorithm based on intracranial eeg and random forest classification. *International Journal of Neural Systems*, 25(05): 1550023, 2015.

[138] Panagiotis Drakopoulos, George Alex Koulieris and Katerina Mania. Front camera eye tracking for mobile vr. In *2020 IEEE Conference on Virtual Reality and 3D User Interfaces Abstracts and Workshops (VRW)*, pp. 642–643, 2020.

[139] Jocelyn Dunstan, Marcela Aguirre, Magdalena Bastías, Claudia Nau, Thomas A Glass et al. Predicting nationwide obesity from food sales using machine learning. *Health Informatics Journal*, 26(1): 652–663, 2020.

[140] Ted Dunstone and Neil Yager. *Biometric System and Data Analysis: Design, Evaluation, and Data Mining*. Springer Science & Business Media, 2008.

[141] Dalila Durães, Davide Carneiro, Javier Bajo and Paulo Novais. Modelling a smart environment for nonintrusive analysis of attention in the workplace. *Expert Systems*, 35(5): e12275, 2018. e12275 EXSY-Jun-17-128.R2.

[142] Ralf Dörner, Stefan Göbel, Wolfgang Effelsberg and Josef Wiemeyer, editors. *Serious Games*. Springer International Publishing, Cham, 2016.

[143] John S Ebersole. Ambulatory cassette eeg. *Journal of Clinical Neurophysiology: Official Publication of the American Electroencephalographic Society*, 2(4): 397–418, 1985.

[144] Kohtaroh Edakawa, Takufumi Yanagisawa, Haruhiko Kishima, Ryohei Fukuma, Satoru Oshino et al. Detection of epileptic seizures using phase–amplitude coupling in intracranial electroencephalography. *Scientific Reports*, 6: 25422, 2016.

[145] Maria Egger, Matthias Ley and Sten Hanke. Emotion recognition from physiological signal analysis: A review. *Electronic Notes in Theoretical Computer Science*, 343: 35–55, 2019. The proceedings of AmI, the 2018 European Conference on Ambient Intelligence.

[146] Alaa El Masri, Harry Wechsler, Peter Likarish and Brent Byung Hoon Kang. Identifying users with application-specific command streams. In *Privacy, Security and Trust (PST), 2014 Twelfth Annual International Conference on*, pp. 232–238. IEEE, 2014.

[147] Hussein El Saadi, Ahmed Farouk Al-Sadek and Mohamed Waleed Fakhr. Informed under-sampling for enhancing patient specific epileptic seizure detection. *International Journal of Computer Applications*, 57(16), 2012.

[148] Abdulmotaleb El Saddik. Digital twins: The convergence of multimedia technologies. *IEEE MultiMedia*, 25(2): 87–92, 2018.

[149] Ayman El-Sayed. Multi-biometric systems: A state of the art survey and research directions. *International Journal of Advanced Computer Science and Applications*, 2015.

[150] Adel S Elmaghraby and Michael M Losavio. Cyber security challenges in smart cities: Safety, security and privacy. *Journal of Advanced Research*, 5(4): 491–497, 2014.

[151] Jerome Engel. A practical guide for routine eeg studies in epilepsy. *Journal of Clinical Neurophysiology*, 1(2): 109–142, 1984.

[152] Jerome Engel Jr. A proposed diagnostic scheme for people with epileptic seizures and with epilepsy: Report of the ilae task force on classification and terminology. *Epilepsia*, 42(6): 796–803, 2001.

[153] Jerome Engel Jr. *Seizures and Epilepsy*, volume 83. Oxford University Press, 2013.

[154] Mohammad Reza Eskandarion, Taghi Golmohamadi, Arash Alipour Tabrizi, Reza Nasr, Mohsen Tabasi et al. Optimizing denaturing hplc as a robust technique for identification of short tandem repeats (str) in forensic medicine. *Journal of Forensic and Legal Medicine*, 61: 108–114, 2019.

[155] Bjoern M Eskofier, Sunghoon Ivan Lee, Manuela Baron, André Simon, Christine F Martindale et al. An overview of smart shoes in the internet of health things: Gait and mobility assessment in health promotion and disease monitoring. *Applied Sciences*, 7(10): 986, 2017.

[156] Brian S Everitt, Sabine Landau, Morven Leese and Daniel Stahl. An introduction to classification and clustering. *Cluster Analysis*, 5: 1–13, 2011.

[157] Luisa Fasulo, Alessandro Naddeo and Nicola Cappetti. A study of classroom seat (dis)comfort: Relationships between body movements, center of pressure on the seat, and lower limbs' sensations. *Applied Ergonomics*, 74: 233–240, 2019.

[158] Howard J Faulkner, Hisatomi Arima and Armin Mohamed. The utility of prolonged outpatient ambulatory eeg. *Seizure*, 21(7): 491–495, 2012.

[159] Marcos Faundez-Zanuy. Signature recognition state-of-the-art. *IEEE Aerospace and Electronic Systems Magazine*, 20(7): 28–32, 2005.

[160] Usama M Fayyad, Gregory Piatetsky-Shapiro, Padhraic Smyth and Ramasamy Uthurusamy. Advances in knowledge discovery and data mining. In *17th Pacific-Asia Conference. American Association for Artificial Intelligence*, 1996.

[161] Paul Fergus, A Hussain, David Hignett, Dhiya Al-Jumeily, Khaled Abdel-Aziz et al. A machine learning system for automated whole-brain seizure detection. *Applied Computing and Informatics*, 12(1): 70–89, 2016.

[162] Salim Ferhat, Christophe Domain, Julien Vidal, Didier Nöel, Bernard Ratier et al. Flexible thermoelectric device based on tis2(ha)x n-type nanocomposite printed on paper. *Organic Electronics*, 68: 256–263, 2019.

[163] Tiago M. Fernández-Caramés and Paula Fraga-Lamas. Towards the internetof-smart-clothing: A review on IoT wearables and garments for creating intelligent connected E-textiles. *Electronics (Switzerland)*, 7(12), 2018.

[164] Colin D Ferrie. Idiopathic generalized epilepsies imitating focal epilepsies. *Epilepsia*, 46: 91–95, 2005.

[165] Kirsten M Fiest, Khara M Sauro, Samuel Wiebe, Scott B Patten, Churl-Su Kwon et al. Prevalence and incidence of epilepsy: A systematic review and meta-analysis of international studies. *Neurology*, 88(3): 296–303, 2017.

[166] Robert S Fisher, J Helen Cross, Carol D'souza, Jacqueline A French, Sheryl R Haut et al. Instruction manual for the ILAE 2017 operational classification of seizure types. *Epilepsia*, 58(4): 531–542, 2017.

[167] Robert S Fisher, J Helen Cross, Carol D'souza, Jacqueline A French, Sheryl R Haut et al. Instruction manual for the ilae 2017 operational classification of seizure types. *Epilepsia*, 58(4): 531–542, 2017.

[168] Eric Flior and Kazimierz Kowalski. Continuous biometric user authentication in online examinations. In *Information Technology: New Generations (ITNG), 2010 Seventh International Conference on*, pp. 488–492. IEEE, 2010.

[169] Epilepsy Foundation. Types of seizures. *Neurology Now*, 4(6): 36, 2008. ISBN: 1800345437.

[170] Epilepsy Foundation. Types of seizures. *Neurology Now*, 4(6): 36, 2008. ISBN: 1800345437.

[171] Andrew M Fraser and Harry L Swinney. Independent coordinates for strange attractors from mutual information. *Physical Review A*, 33(2): 1134, 1986.

[172] Sigfredo Fuentes, Eden Tongson and Claudia Gonzalez Viejo. Novel digital technologies implemented in sensory science and consumer perception. *Current Opinion in Food Science*, 41: 99–106, 2021.

[173] Daniel Fuller, Emily Colwell, Jonathan Low, Kassia Orychock, Melissa Tobin et al. Reliability and validity of commercially available wearable devices for measuring steps, energy expenditure, and heart rate: A systematic review (preprint). *JMIR mHealth and uHealth*, 8: 03 2020.

[174] G Bourhis, K Moumen, P Pino, S Rohmer and A Pruski. Assisted navigation for a powered wheelchair. In *Proceedings of IEEE Systems Man and Cybernetics Conference—SMC*, volume 3, pp. 553–558 vol. 3, October 1993. Journal Abbreviation: Proceedings of IEEE Systems Man and Cybernetics Conference - SMC.

[175] G Jang, J Kim, S Lee and Y Choi. EMG-based continuous control scheme with simple classifier for electric-powered wheelchair. *IEEE Transactions on Industrial Electronics*, 63(6): 3695–3705, June 2016.

[176] Christopher Gaffney and Cerianne Robertson. Smarter than smart: Rio de Janeiro's flawed emergence as a smart city. *Journal of Urban Technology*, 25(3): 47–64, 2018.

[177] Davrondzhon Gafurov, Kirsi Helkala and Torkjel Søndrol. Biometric gait authentication using accelerometer sensor. *JCP*, 1(7): 51–59, 2006.

[178] Mikel Galar, Alberto Fernandez, Edurne Barrenechea, Humberto Bustince, and Francisco Herrera. A review on ensembles for the class imbalance problem: bagging-, boosting-, and hybrid-based approaches. *IEEE Transactions on Systems, Man, and Cybernetics, Part C (Applications and Reviews)*, 42(4): 463–484, 2011.

[179] Ravil R Garafutdinov, Assol R Sakhabutdinova, Petr A Slominsky, Farit G Aminev and Alexey V. Chemeris. A new digital approach to snp encoding for dna identification. *Forensic Science International*, 317: 110520, 2020.

[180] Crispin W Gardiner. *Stochastic Methods: A Handbook for the Natural and Social Sciences*. Springer, 2009.

[181] Vikas Garg, Abhishek Singhal and Pooja Tiwari. A study on transformation in technological based biometrics attendance system: Human resource management practice. In *2018 8th International Conference on Cloud Computing, Data Science Engineering (Confluence)*, pp. 809–813, 2018.

[182] Isabelle Gaudet, Alejandra Hüsser, Phetsamone Vannasing and Anne Gallagher. Functional brain connectivity of language functions in children revealed by eeg and meg: A systematic review. *Frontiers in Human Neuroscience*, 14: 62, 2020.

[183] M Gayathri, C Malathy and M Prabhakaran. A review on various biometric techniques, its features, methods, security issues and application areas. pp. 931–941. *In*: S Smys, João Manuel RS Tavares, Valentina Emilia Balas and Abdullah M Iliyasu, editors, (eds.). *Computational Vision and Bio-Inspired Computing*, Cham, 2020. Springer International Publishing.

[184] Peyvand Ghaderyan, Ataollah Abbasi and Mohammad Hossein Sedaaghi. An efficient seizure prediction method using knn-based undersampling and linear frequency measures. *Journal of Neuroscience Methods*, 232: 134–142, 2014.

[185] Frederic A Gibbs. Electroencephalography in epilepsy. *The Journal of Pediatrics*, 15(6): 749–762, 1939.

[186] Mark Glantz. Internet radio adopts a human touch: A study of 12 streaming music services. *Journal of Radio & Audio Media*, 23(1): 36–49, 2016.

[187] John Gleaves. Biometrics and antidoping enforcement in professional sport. *The American Journal of Bioethics*, 17(1): 77–79, 2017.

[188] A. Godfrey. Wearables for independent living in older adults: Gait and falls. *Maturitas*, 100: 16–26, 2017.

[189] Parnaz Golnar-Nik, Sajjad Farashi and Mir-Shahram Safari. The application of eeg power for the prediction and interpretation of consumer decision making: A neuromarketing study. *Physiology & Behavior*, 207: 90–98, 2019.

[190] MJ Goodwin, DA Sanders, GA Poland and IJ Stott. Navigational assistance for disabled wheelchair-users. *Journal of Systems Architecture*, 43(1): 73–79, March 1997.

[191] Mark A Gorski, Stanley M Mimoto, Vivek Khare, Viprali Bhatkar and Arthur H Combs. Real-time digital biometric monitoring during elite athletic competition: sSystem feasibility with awearable medical-grade sensor. *Digital Biomarkers*, 5(1): 37–43, 2021.

[192] Peter Grassberger and Itamar Procaccia. Characterization of strange attractors. *Physical Review Letters*, 50(5): 346, 1983.

[193] JH Gruzelier, M Foks, T Steffert, MJ-L Chen and T Ros. Beneficial outcome from eeg-neurofeedback on creative music performance, attention and well-being in school children. *Biological Psychology*, 95: 86–95, 2014. SAN (Society of Applied Neuroscience) Special issue on Neurofeedback.

[194] Carlos AM Guerreiro, Maria Augusta Montenegro, Eliane Kobayashi, Ana Lúcia A Noronha, Marilisa M Guerreiro et al. Daytime outpatient versus inpatient video-eeg monitoring for presurgical evaluation in temporal lobe epilepsy. *Journal of Clinical Neurophysiology*, 19(3): 204–208, 2002.

[195] Oana Gurau, William J Bosl and Charles R Newton. How useful is electroencephalography in the diagnosis of autism spectrum disorders and the delineation of subtypes: A systematic review. *Frontiers in Psychiatry*, 8: 121, 2017.

[196] John Guttag, Ali Shoeb, Blaise Bourgeois, S Treves, Steven Schachter et al. Patient-specific seizure onset detection system, 2006. US Patent App. 11/140,551.

[197] Hadi Habibzadeh, Tolga Soyata, Burak Kantarci, Azzedine Boukerche and Cem Kaptan. Sensing, communication and security planes: A new challenge for a smart city system design. *Computer Networks*, 144: 163–200, 2018.

[198] Shahab Haghayegh, Sepideh Khoshnevis, Michael H Smolensky, Kenneth R Diller and Richard J Castriotta. Accuracy of wrist band fitbit models in assessing sleep: Systematic review and meta-analysis. *J Med Internet Res*, 21(11): e16273, Nov 2019.

[199] Adam Hakim and Dino J Levy. A gateway to consumers' minds: Achievements, caveats, and prospects of electroencephalography-based prediction in neuromarketing. *WIREs Cognitive Science*, 10(2): e1485, 2019.

[200] Naser Hakimi, Ata Jodeiri, Mahya Mirbagheri and S Kamaledin Setarehdan. Proposing a convolutional neural network for stress assessment by means of derived heart rate from functional near infrared spectroscopy. *Computers in Biology and Medicine*, 121: 103810, 2020.

[201] Mark Hall, Eibe Frank, Geoffrey Holmes, Bernhard Pfahringer, Peter Reutemann et al. The weka data mining software: Aan update. *ACM SIGKDD Eexplorations Newsletter*, 11(1): 10–18, 2009.

[202] Omar Hamdy and Issa Traoré. Cognitive-based biometrics system for static user authentication. In *Internet Monitoring and Protection, 2009. ICIMP '09. Fourth International Conference on,* pp. 90–97. IEEE, 2009.

[203] Nicolas Hamelin, Park Thaichon, Christopher Abraham, Nicholas Driver, Joe Lipscombe et al. Storytelling, the scale of persuasion and retention: A neuromarketing approach. *Journal of Retailing and Consumer Services,* 55: 102099, 2020.

[204] Ajna Hamidovic, Kathryne Van Hedger, So Hee Choi, Stephanie Flowers, Margaret Wardle et al. Quantitative meta-analysis of heart rate variability finds reduced parasympathetic cardiac tone in women compared to men during laboratory-based social stress. *Neuroscience & Biobehavioral Reviews,* 114: 194–200, 2020.

[205] N Hammond. Tonic–clonic seizures. In *Reference Module in Biomedical Sciences.* Elsevier, 2016.

[206] Dong-Kyoon Han, Jong-Myoung Kim, Eun-Jong Cha and Tae-Soo Lee. Wheelchair type biomedical system with event-recorder function. *Conference proceedings: Annual International Conference of the IEEE Engineering in Medicine and Biology Society. IEEE Engineering in Medicine and Biology Society. Annual Conference,* 2008: 1435–1438, 2008. Place: United States.

[207] Jiawei Han, Micheline Kamber and Jian Pei. Data mining concepts and techniques third edition. *The Morgan Kaufmann Series in Data Management Systems,* pp. 83–124, 2011.

[208] Shunjie Han, Cao Qubo and Han Meng. Parameter selection in svm with rbf kernel function. In *World Automation Congress 2012,* pp. 1–4. IEEE, 2012.

[209] Gerhard P Hancke, Bruno De Carvalho e Silva and Gerhard P Hancke, Jr. The role of advanced sensing in smart cities. *Sensors,* 13(1): 393–425, 2013.

[210] J Hanley. Telemetry in health care. *Biomedical Engineering,* 11(8): 269–272, 1976.

[211] Bhanwala Harender and RK Sharma. Dwt based epileptic seizure detection from eeg signal using k-nn classifier. In *2017 International Conference Trends in Electronics and Informatics (ICEI),* pp. 762–765. IEEE, 2017.

[212] Bilal Hassan, Ebroul Izquierdo and Tomas Piatrik. Soft biometrics: A survey. *Multimedia Tools and Applications,* pp. 1–44, 2021.

[213] Jigna J Hathaliya, Sudeep Tanwar, Sudhanshu Tyagi and Neeraj Kumar. Securing electronics healthcare records in healthcare 4.0: A biometric-based approach. *Computers & Electrical Engineering*, 76: 398–410, 2019.

[214] Hauser and Beghi. Nombre articulo. In *Nombre Proceedintw*, page Paginas, 2008.

[215] Gabriel Hermosilla, Javier Ruiz del Solar, Rodrigo Verschae and Mauricio Correa. A comparative study of thermal face recognition methods in unconstrained environments. *Pattern Recognition*, 45(7): 2445–2459, 2012.

[216] Christoph S Herrmann, Daniel Strüber, Randolph F Helfrich and Andreas K Engel. Eeg oscillations: from correlation to causality. *International Journal of Psychophysiology*, 103: 12–21, 2016.

[217] Tosca-Marie Heunis, Chris Aldrich and Petrus J de Vries. Recent advances in resting-state electroencephalography biomarkers for autism spectrum disorder—A review of methodological and clinical challenges. *Pediatric Neurology*, 61: 28–37, 2016.

[218] Desmond J Higham and Nicholas J Higham. *MATLAB guide*. SIAM, 2016.

[219] Darren C Hill, Shruti Sudhakar, Christopher S Hill, Tonya S King, Ingrid U Scott et al. Intraoperative aberrometry versus preoperative biometry for intraocular lens power selection in axial myopia. *Journal of Cataract and Refractive Surgery*, 43(4): 505–510, 2017.

[220] Tin Kam Ho. The random subspace method for constructing decision forests. *IEEE Transactions on Pattern Analysis and Machine Intelligence*, 20(8): 832–844, 1998.

[221] Hwei P Hsu. *Schaum's Outline of Theory and Problems of Probability, Random Variables, and Random Processes*. McGraw-Hill, 1997.

[222] John R Hughes. Eeg in clinical practice, 1994.

[223] Hugo López-Gatell Ramírez on Twitter. Available at https://twitter.com/HLGatell/status/1318346231408599040 (accessed: 2020-10-20).

[224] Samir Huseynov, Bachir Kassas, Michelle S Segovia and Marco A Palma. Incorporating biometric data in models of consumer choice. *Applied Economics*, 51(14): 1514–1531, 2019.

[225] Shaun A Hussain, Raymond Zhou, Catherine Jacobson, Julius Weng, Emily Cheng et al. Perceived efficacy of cannabidiol-enriched cannabis

extracts for treatment of pediatric epilepsy: A potential role for infantile spasms and lennox–gastaut syndrome. *Epilepsy & Behavior*, 47: 138–141, 2015.

[226] Hyunwoo Hwangbo, Yang Sok Kim and Kyung Jin Cha. Use of the smart store for persuasive marketing and immersive customer experiences: A case study of korean apparel enterprise. *Mobile Information Systems*, 2017: 4738340, Mar 2017.

[227] Matthias Ihle, Hinnerk Feldwisch-Drentrup, César A Teixeira, Adrien Witon, Björn Schelter et al. EPILEPSIAE–a european epilepsy database. *Computer Methods and Programs in Biomedicine*, 106(3): 127–138, 2012.

[228] Celestine Iwendi, Ali Kashif Bashir, Atharva Peshkar, R Sujatha, Jyotir Moy Chatterjee et al. Covid-19 patient health prediction using boosted random forest algorithm. *Frontiers in Public Health*, 8: 357, 2020.

[229] J Ahmad, H Andersson and J Sidén. Screen-printed piezoresistive sensors for monitoring pressure distribution in wheelchair. *IEEE Sensors Journal*, 19(6): 2055–2063, March 2019.

[230] Jesse V Jacobs, Lawrence J Hettinger, Yueng-Hsiang Huang, Susan Jeffries, Mary F Lesch et al. Employee acceptance of wearable technology in the workplace. *Applied Ergonomics*, 78: 148–156, 2019.

[231] Katja Lindskov Jacobsen. On humanitarian refugee biometrics and new forms of intervention. *Journal of Intervention and Statebuilding*, 11(4): 529–551, 2017.

[232] Anil K Jain, Patrick Flynn and Arun A Ross. *Handbook of Biometrics*. Springer Science & Business Media, 2007.

[233] Anil K Jain, Patrick Flynn and Arun A Ross. *Handbook of Biometrics*. Springer Science & Business Media, 2007.

[234] Anil K Jain and Ajay Kumar. Biometrics of next generation: An overview. *Second Generation Biometrics*, 12(1): 2–3, 2010.

[235] Gareth James, Daniela Witten, Trevor Hastie and Robert Tibshirani. *An Introduction to Statistical Learning*, volume 103 of *Springer Texts in Statistics*. Springer New York, New York, NY, 2013.

[236] Herbert H Jasper and Ira C Nichols. Electrical signs of cortical function in epilepsy and allied disorders. *American Journal of Psychiatry*, 94(4): 835–851, 1938.

[237] Byoungjun Jeon, Boseong Jeong, Seunghoon Jee, Yan Huang, Youngmin Kim et al. A facial recognition mobile app for patient safety and biometric identification: Design, development, and validation. *JMIR mHealth and uHealth*, 7(4): e11472, April 2019.

[238] Shafali S Jeste, Joel Frohlich and Sandra K Loo. Electrophysiological biomarkers of diagnosis and outcome in neurodevelopmental disorders. *Current Opinion in Neurology*, 28(2): 110, 2015.

[239] Ping Jiang, Jonathan Winkley, Can Zhao, Robert Munnoch, Geyong Min et al. An intelligent information forwarder for healthcare big data systems with distributed wearable sensors. *IEEE Systems Journal*, 10(3): 1147–1159, 2016.

[240] Xiao Jiang, Gui-Bin Bian and Zean Tian. Removal of artifacts from eeg signals: A review. *Sensors*, 19(5): 987, 2019.

[241] Rozmin Jiwani, Brittany Dennis, Chandler Bess, Siler Monk, Kylie Meyer et al. Assessing acceptability and patient experience of a behavioral lifestyle intervention using fitbit technology in older adults to manage type 2 diabetes amid covid-19 pandemic: A focus group study. *Geriatric Nursing*, 42(1): 57–64, 2021.

[242] Hajer Jomaa, Rostom Mabrouk and Nawres Khlifa. Validation of iterative multi-resolution method for partial volume correction and quantification improvement in pet image. *Biomedical Signal Processing and Control*, 60: 101954, 2020.

[243] Damon Jones, David Molitor and Julian Reif. What do workplace wellness programs do? Evidence from the Illinois Wworkplace wellness study. *The Quarterly Journal of Economics*, 134(4): 1747–1791, Nov 2019.

[244] Jin Ju, Yunhee Shin and Eun Kim. Vision based interface system for hands free control of an intelligent wheelchair. *Journal of NeuroEngineering and Rehabilitation*, 6(1): 33, 2009.

[245] Felix Juefei-Xu and Marios Savvides. Unconstrained periocular biometric acquisition and recognition using cots ptz camera for uncooperative and noncooperative subjects. In *2012 IEEE Workshop on the Applications of Computer Vision (WACV)*, pp. 201–208. IEEE, 2012.

[246] David Juárez-Varón, Victoria Tur-Viñes, Alejandro Rabasa-Dolado and Kristina Polotskaya. An adaptive machine learning methodology applied to neuromarketing analysis: Prediction of consumer behaviour regarding

the key elements of the packaging design of an educational toy. *Social Sciences*, 9(9), 2020.

[247] Bharath Kumar KK, Sudha Mani Ch., Naqi Mohd Abdul and Sireesha Pendem. Smart jacket for health monitoring using labview. *Materials Today: Proceedings*, 2020.

[248] K Maatoug, M Njah and M Jallouli. Electric wheelchair trajectory tracking control based on fuzzy logic controller. In *2019 19th International Conference on Sciences and Techniques of Automatic Control and Computer Engineering (STA)*, pp. 191–195, March 2019. Journal Abbreviation: 2019 19th International Conference on Sciences and Techniques of Automatic Control and Computer Engineering (STA).

[249] K Nakajima and K Sasaki. Personal recognition using head-top image for health-monitoring system in the home. In *The 26th Annual International Conference of the IEEE Engineering in Medicine and Biology Society*, volume 2, pp. 3147–3150, September 2004. Journal Abbreviation: The 26th Annual International Conference of the IEEE Engineering in Medicine and Biology Society.

[250] C Kabdebon, François Leroy, H Simmonet, Matthieu Perrot, Jessica Dubois et al. Anatomical correlations of the international 10–20 sensor placement system in infants. *Neuroimage*, 99: 342–356, 2014.

[251] Alper Kanak and Ibrahim Sogukpinar. Biotam: A technology acceptance model for biometric authentication systems. *IET Biometrics*, 6(6): 457–467, 2017.

[252] Burak Kantarci, Melike Erol-Kantarci and Stephanie Schuckers. Towards secure cloud-centric internet of biometric things. In *2015 IEEE 4th International Conference on Cloud Networking (CloudNet)*, pp. 81–83, 2015.

[253] Katrina Karkazis and Jennifer R Fishman. Tracking U.S. Professional Athletes: The Ethics of Biometric Technologies. *The American Journal of Bioethics: AJOB*, 17(1): 45–60, Jan 2017.

[254] Judy Keenan and Kimberly Barnhart. Development of yes/no systems in individuals with severe traumatic brain injuries. *Augmentative and Alternative Communication*, 9(3): 184–190, 1993.

[255] Sarah A Kelley and Eric H Kossoff. Doose syndrome (myoclonic–astatic epilepsy): 40 years of progress. *Developmental Medicine & Child Neurology*, 52(11): 988–993, 2010.

[256] Matthew B Kennel, Reggie Brown and Henry DI Abarbanel. Determining embedding dimension for phase-space reconstruction using a geometrical construction. *Physical Review A*, 45(6): 3403, 1992.

[257] Alaa Kharbouch, Ali Shoeb, John Guttag and Sydney S Cash. An algorithm for seizure onset detection using intracranial eeg. *Epilepsy & Behavior*, 22: S29–S35, 2011.

[258] Pyoung Won Kim. Ambient intelligence in a smart classroom for assessing students' engagement levels. *Journal of Ambient Intelligence and Humanized Computing*, 10(10): 3847–3852, Oct 2019.

[259] Sang Bin Kim, Sin Jae Lee and Jung Hyun Han. Stretcharms: Promoting stretching exercise with a smartwatch. *International Journal of Human–Computer Interaction*, 34(3): 218–225, 2018.

[260] Wiltold Kinsner. Towards evolving symbiotic education based on digital twins. *Mondo Digitale*, 18(80), 2019.

[261] Lech Kipiński, Reinhard König, Cezary Sielużycki and Wojciech Kordecki. Application of modern tests for stationarity to single-trial meg data. *Biological Cybernetics*, 105(3): 183–195, 2011.

[262] Jessica Sofranko Kisenwether and Robert T Sataloff. The effect of microphone type on acoustical measures of synthesized vowels. *Journal of Voice*, 29(5): 548–551, 2015.

[263] Wai Kit Cheng, Ho Lok Lam, Fei Lin and Ming Ge. A customizable smart shoes with location tracking function for the elderly. *Materials Today: Proceedings*, 16: 1423–1430, 2019. Shape Memory Applications, Research and Technology 2018.

[264] Wolfgang Klimesch. An algorithm for the eeg frequency architecture of consciousness and brain body coupling. *Frontiers in Human Neuroscience*, 7: 766, 2013.

[265] Wolfgang Klimesch. The frequency architecture of brain and brain body oscillations: An analysis. *European Journal of Neuroscience*, 48(7): 2431–2453, 2018.

[266] Marek Klonowski, Marcin Plata and Piotr Syga. User authorization based on hand geometry without special equipment. *Pattern Recognition*, 73: 189–201, 2018.

[267] Reinmar J Kobler, Andreea I Sburlea, Valeria Mondini and Gernot R Müller-Putz. Hear to remove pops and drifts: the high-variance electrode

artifact removal (hear) algorithm. In *2019 41st Annual International Conference of the IEEE Engineering in Medicine and Biology Society (EMBC)*, pp. 5150–5155. IEEE, 2019.

[268] Otilia Kocsis, Aris Lalos, Gerasimos Arvanitis and Konstantinos Moustakas. Multi-model short-term prediction schema for mhealth empowering asthma self-management. *Electronic Notes in Theoretical Computer Science*, 343: 3–17, 2019. The Proceedings of AmI, the 2018 European Conference on Ambient Intelligence.

[269] Chorng-Shiuh Koong, Tzu-I Yang and Chien-Chao Tseng. A user authentication scheme using physiological and behavioral biometrics for multitouch devices. *The Scientific World Journal*, 2014, 2014.

[270] MB Korsakova, AB Kozlova, NA Arkhipova, LV Shishkina, PA Vlasov et al. Features of ictal and interictal electrical activity in assessment of the epileptogenic zone in children with focal cortical dysplasias. *Burdenko's Journal of Neurosurgery*, 68, 2019.

[271] Anton Kos and Anton Umek. Wearable sensor devices for prevention and rehabilitation in healthcare: Swimming exercise with real-time therapist feedback. *IEEE Internet of Things Journal*, 6(2): 1331–1341, 2019.

[272] Sotiris B Kotsiantis, I Zaharakis and P Pintelas. Supervised machine learning: A review of classification techniques. *Emerging Artificial Intelligence Applications in Computer Engineering*, 160(1): 3–24, 2007.

[273] Mark A Kramer, Eric D Kolaczyk and Heidi E Kirsch. Emergent network topology at seizure onset in humans. *Epilepsy Research*, 79(2-3): 173–186, 2008.

[274] Oliver Kramer. *Dimensionality Reduction with Unsupervised Nearest Neighbors*. Springer, 2013.

[275] Niranjana Krupa, Karthik Anantharam, Manoj Sanker, Sameer Datta and John Vijay Sagar. Recognition of emotions in autistic children using physiological signals. *Health and Technology*, 6(2): 137–147, 2016.

[276] Parag Kulkarni and Tim Farnham. Smart city wireless connectivity considerations and cost analysis: Lessons learnt from smart water case studies. *IEEE Access*, 4(c): 660–672, 2016.

[277] Ashutosh Kumar, Roshan Bharti, Deepak Gupta and Anish Kumar Saha. Improvement in boosting method by using rustboost technique for class imbalanced data. In *Recent Developments in Machine Learning and Data Analytics*, pp. 51–66. Springer, 2019.

[278] Jae Young Kwon, Min-Tae Jeon, Un Ju Jung, Dong Woon Kim, Gyeong Joon Moon et al. Perspective: Therapeutic potential of flavonoids as alternative medicines in epilepsy. *Advances in Nutrition*, 10(5): 778–790, 2019.

[279] Sina Mansour L, Ye Tian, BT Thomas Yeo, Vanessa Cropley and Andrew Zalesky. High-resolution connectomic fingerprints: Mapping neural identity and behavior. *NeuroImage*, 229: 117695, 2021.

[280] L Yang, Y Ge, W Li, W Rao and W Shen. A home mobile healthcare system for wheelchair users. In *Proceedings of the 2014 IEEE 18th International Conference on Computer Supported Cooperative Work in Design (CSCWD)*, pp. 609–614, May 2014. Journal Abbreviation: Proceedings of the 2014 IEEE 18th International Conference on Computer Supported Cooperative Work in Design (CSCWD).

[281] Ruggero Donida Labati, Angelo Genovese, Enrique Muñoz, Vincenzo Piuri, Fabio Scotti et al. Computational intelligence for biometric applications: A survey. *International Journal of Computing*, 15(1): 40–49, 2016.

[282] Terrence D Lagerlund, Frank W Sharbrough, Clifford R Jack Jr, Bradley J Erickson, Dan C Strelow et al. Determination of 10–20 system electrode locations using magnetic resonance image scanning with markers. *Electroencephalography and Clinical Neurophysiology*, 86(1): 7–14, 1993.

[283] Thomas N Lal, Thilo Hinterberger, Guido Widman, Michael Schröder, N Jeremy Hill et al. Methods towards invasive human brain computer interfaces. In *Advances in Neural Information Processing Systems*, pp. 737–744, 2005.

[284] Rachel Lampert. Ecg signatures of psychological stress. *Journal of Electrocardiology*, 48(6): 1000–1005, 2015.

[285] Andreas D Landmark and Børge Sjøbakk. Tracking customer behaviour in fashion retail using rfid. *International Journal of Retail & Distribution Management*, 45(7/8): 844–858, Jan 2017.

[286] Oscar D Lara and Miguel A Labrador. A survey on human activity recognition using wearable sensors. *IEEE Communications Surveys & Tutorials*, 15(3): 1192–1209, 2012.

[287] Alex Lau-Zhu, Michael PH Lau and Gráinne McLoughlin. Mobile eeg in research on neurodevelopmental disorders: Opportunities and challenges. *Developmental Cognitive nNeuroscience*, 36: 100635, 2019.

[288] Andrew Lawley, Shaun Evans, Francesco Manfredonia and Andrea E Cavanna. The role of outpatient ambulatory electroencephalography in the diagnosis and management of adults with epilepsy or nonepileptic attack disorder: A systematic literature review. *Epilepsy & Behavior*, 53: 26–30, 2015.

[289] Dung Le, Marlene Pratt, Ying Wang, Noel Scott and Gui Lohmann. How to win the consumer's heart? Exploring appraisal determinants of consumer pre-consumption emotions. *International Journal of Hospitality Management*, 88: 102542, 2020.

[290] Sandra Leaton Gray. Biometrics in schools. pp. 405–424. *In*: Jo Deakin, Emmeline Taylor and Aaron Kupchik (eds.). *The Palgrave International Handbook of School Discipline, Surveillance, and Social Control*. Springer International Publishing, Cham, 2018.

[291] XK Lee, NI Chee, J Ong, Teck Boon Teo, Elaine van Rijn et al. Validation of a consumer sleep wearable device with actigraphy and polysomnography in adolescents across sleep opportunity manipulations. *Journal of Clinical Sleep Medicine: JCSM: Official Publication of the American Academy of Sleep Medicine*, 2019.

[292] Yung-Li Lee, Jwo Pan, Richard Hathaway and Mark Barkey. *Fatigue tTesting and Analysis: Theory and Practice*, volume 13. Butterworth-Heinemann, 2005.

[293] Agatha Lenartowicz and Sandra K Loo. Use of eeg to diagnose adhd. *Current Psychiatry Reports*, 16(11): 498, 2014.

[294] Andrew C Leon, Lori L Davis and Helena C Kraemer. The role and interpretation of pilot studies in clinical research. *Journal of Psychiatric Research*, 45(5): 626–629, 2011.

[295] Soren Leth, John Hansen, Olav W Nielsen and Birthe Dinesen. Evaluation of commercial self-monitoring devices for clinical purposes: Results from the future patient trial, phase i. *Sensors*, 17(1), 2017.

[296] Crockett, LH, Elliot, RA, Enderwitz, MA and Stewart, R. *The Zynq Book*. University of Strathclyde, 2014.

[297] Meijing Li, Xiuming Yu, Keun Ryu, Sanghyuk Lee and Nipon Theera-Umpon. Face recognition technology development with gabor, pca and svm methodology under illumination normalization condition. *Cluster Computing*, 21, 03 2018.

[298] Ming-ai Li, Hai-na Liu, Wei Zhu and Jin-fu Yang. Applying improved multiscale fuzzy entropy for feature extraction of mi-eeg. *Applied Sciences*, 7(1): 92, 2017.

[299] Ryan T Li, Scott R Kling, Michael J Salata, Sean A Cupp, Joseph Sheehan et al. Wearable performance devices in sports medicine. *Sports Health*, 8(1): 74–78, 2016.

[300] Yan Li, Peng Paul Wen et al. Clustering technique-based least square support vector machine for eeg signal classification. *Computer Methods and Programs in Biomedicine*, 104(3): 358–372, 2011.

[301] Yang Li, Wenming Zheng, Zhen Cui and Tong Zhang. Face recognition based on recurrent regression neural network. *Neurocomputing*, 297: 50–58, 2018.

[302] Tan Lii Inn. Smart City Technologies Take on Covid-19—Penang Institute, March 2020.

[303] Chin-Teng Lin, Li-Wei Ko, Meng-Hsiu Chang, Jeng-Ren Duann, Jing-Ying Chen et al. Review of wireless and wearable electroencephalogram systems and brain-computer interfaces—a mini-review. *Gerontology*, 56(1): 112–119, 2010.

[304] David J Livingstone. *Artificial Neural Networks: Methods and Applications*. Springer, 2008.

[305] Erik K St Louis, LC Frey, JW Britton, JL Hopp, PJ Korb et al. Electroencephalography (eeg): An introductory text and atlas of normal and abnormal findings in adults. *Children, and Infants*, 2016.

[306] Lovisotto Giulio, Malik Raghav, Sluganovic Ivo, Roeschlin Marc, Trueman Paul et al. Mobile biometrics in financial services: A five factor framework. University of Oxford. Available at https://www.cs.ox.ac.uk/files/9113/Mobile%20Biometrics%20in%20Financial%20Services.pdf (accessed: 2021-05-11), 2017.

[307] David Lowrence. Biometrics and retail: Moving towards the future. *Biometric Technology Today*, 2014(2): 7–9, 2014.

[308] Jorge de J Lozoya-Santos, Victorino Sepúlveda-Arróniz, Juan C Tudon-Martinez and Ricardo A Ramirez-Mendoza. Survey on biometry for cognitive automotive systems. *Cognitive Systems Research*, 55: 175–191, 2019.

[309] Jing Luan, Zhong Yao, Fu Tao Zhao and Hao Liu. Search product and experience product online reviews: An eye-tracking study on consumers' review search behavior. *Computers in Human Behavior*, 65: 420–430, 2016.

[310] Steven J Luck and Emily S Kappenman. *The Oxford Handbook of Event Related Potential Components.* Oxford University Press, 2011.

[311] Xiaohua Luo, Kougen Zheng, Yunhe Pan and Zhaohui Wu. A tcp/ip implementation for wireless sensor networks. In *IEEE International Conference on Systems, Man and Cybernetics*, 7: 6081–6086, 2004.

[312] Martin Lutz. Non-adhärenz: klinische erfahrung bestätigt, 2016.

[313] MA Eid, N Giakoumidis and A El Saddik. A novel eye-gaze-controlled wheelchair system for navigating unknown environments: Case study with a person with ALS. *IEEE Access*, 4: 558–573, 2016.

[314] M Craciunescu, D Baicu, M Cîrciumaru, S Mocanu and R Dobrescu. Towards the development of autonomous wheelchair. In *2019 22nd International Conference on Control Systems and Computer Science (CSCS)*, pp. 552–557, May 2019. Journal Abbreviation: 2019 22nd International Conference on Control Systems and Computer Science (CSCS).

[315] M Hashimoto, K Takahashi and M Shimada. Wheelchair control using an EOG- and EMG-based gesture interface. In *2009 IEEE/ASME International Conference on Advanced Intelligent Mechatronics*, pp. 1212–1217, July 2009. Journal Abbreviation: 2009 IEEE/ASME International Conference on Advanced Intelligent Mechatronics.

[316] MS Hossain and G Muhammad. Cloud-assisted framework for health monitoring. In *2015 IEEE 28th Canadian Conference on Electrical and Computer Engineering (CCECE)*, pp. 1199–1202, May 2015. Journal Abbreviation: 2015 IEEE 28th Canadian Conference on Electrical and Computer Engineering (CCECE).

[317] Congcong Ma, Wenfeng Li, Raffaele Gravina, Jingjing Cao, Qimeng Li et al. Activity level assessment using a smart cushion for people with a sedentary lifestyle. *Sensors (Basel, Switzerland)*, 17(10), October 2017.

[318] Ioannis Maghiros, Yves Punie, Sabine Delaitre, Elsa Lignos, Carlos Rodriguez et al. Biometrics at the frontiers: Assessing the impact on society. Technical report, Directorate-General for Energy and Transport, European Commission, 2005.

[319] Raju Maharjan, Per Bækgaard and Jakob E. Bardram. Hear me out: Smart speaker based conversational agent to monitor symptoms in mental health. In *Adjunct Proceedings of the 2019 ACM International Joint Conference on Pervasive and Ubiquitous Computing and Proceedings of the 2019 ACM International Symposium on Wearable Computers*, UbiComp/ISWC'19 adjunct, pp. 929–933, New York, NY, USA, 2019. Association for Computing Machinery. Number of pages: 5 Place: London, United Kingdom.

[320] Musa Mahmood, Deogratias Mzurikwao, Yun-Soung Kim, Yongkuk Lee, Saswat Mishra et al. Fully portable and wireless universal brain–machine interfaces enabled by flexible scalp electronics and deep learning algorithm. *Nature Machine Intelligence*, 1(9): 412–422, 2019.

[321] Vladimir A Maksimenko, Sabrina van Heukelum, Vladimir V Makarov, Janita Kelderhuis, Annika Lüttjohann et al. Absence seizure control by a brain computer interface. *Scientific Reports*, 7(1): 1–8, 2017.

[322] Amirsalar Mansouri, Sanjay P Singh and Khalid Sayood. Online eeg seizure detection and localization. *Algorithms*, 12(9): 176, 2019.

[323] Gian Luca Marcialis, Paolo Mastinu and Fabio Roli. Serial fusion of multimodal biometric systems. In *2010 IEEE Workshop on Biometric Measurements and Systems for Security and Medical Applications*, 1–7, 2010.

[324] Dana Marohn. Biometrics in healthcare. *Biometric Technology Today*, 14(9): 9–11, 2006.

[325] Maria De Marsico, Alfredo Petrosino and Stefano Ricciardi. Iris recognition through machine learning techniques: A survey. *Pattern Recognition Letters*, 82: 106–115, 2016. An insight on eye biometrics.

[326] Ramón Martínez-Cancino, Arnaud Delorme, Dung Truong, Fiorenzo Artoni, Kenneth Kreutz-Delgado et al. The open eeglab portal interface: High performance computing with eeglab. *NeuroImage*, 116778, 2020.

[327] Mario Martínez-Galdámez, Jorge Galván Fernández, Miguel Schüller Arteaga, Lorenzo Pérez-Sünchez, Juan F Arenillas et al. Smart glasses evaluation during the covid-19 pandemic: first-use on neurointerventional procedures. Clinical Neurology and Neurosurgery, 106655, 2021.

[328] Michael Massoomi and Eileen Handberg. Increasing and evolving role of smart devices in modern medicine. *European Cardiology Review*, 14: 181–186, 12 2019.

[329] Mathworks. Model-based design for embedded control software development. https://www.mathworks.com/content/dam/mathworks/ mathworksdot-com/campaigns/portals/files/adopting-model-based-design/why-adoptmodel-based-design-for-embedded-control-software-development.pdf (accessed: 2021-05-11), 2021.

[330] Ujjwal Maulik and Sanghamitra Bandyopadhyay. Genetic algorithm-based clustering technique. *Pattern Recognition*, 33(9): 1455–1465, 2000.

[331] Thomas Mayer. Treat epilepsy with cannabis. *DNP-The Neurologist & Psychiatrist*, 21(1): 40–49, 2020.

[332] Luis Carlos Mayor, Jorge Burneo and Juan Ochoa. *Manual de electroencefalografía: Handbook of Electroencephalography*. Ediciones Uniandes-Universidad de los Andes, 2013.

[333] Luis Mañas-Viniegra, Patricia Núñez-Gómez and Victoria Tur-Viñes. Neuromarketing as a strategic tool for predicting how instagramers have an influence on the personal identity of adolescents and young people in spain. *Heliyon*, 6(3): e03578, 2020.

[334] Caroline K Mbuba, Anthony K Ngugi, Charles R Newton and Julie A Carter. The epilepsy treatment gap in developing countries: A systematic review of the magnitude, causes, and intervention strategies. *Epilepsia*, 49(9): 1491–1503, 2008.

[335] Erica D McKenzie, Andrew SP Lim, Edward CW Leung, Andrew J Cole, Alice D Lam et al. Validation of a smartphone-based eeg among people with epilepsy: A prospective study. *Scientific Reports*, 7(1): 1–8, 2017.

[336] Amy McTague and J Helen Cross. Treatment of epileptic encephalopathies. *CNS Drugs*, 27(3): 175–184, 2013.

[337] Daryush D Mehta, Matías Zañartu, Shengran W Feng, Harold A 2nd Cheyne and Robert E Hillman. Mobile voice health monitoring using a wearable accelerometer sensor and a smartphone platform. *IEEE Transactions on Bio-medical Engineering*, 59(11): 3090–3096, November 2012.

[338] Mario Merone, Paolo Soda, Mario Sansone and Carlo Sansone. Ecg databases for biometric systems: A systematic review. *Expert Systems with Applications*, 67: 189–202, 2017.

[339] Antonio Mileti, Gianluigi Guido and M Irene Prete. Nanomarketing: A new frontier for neuromarketing. *Psychology & Marketing*, 33(8): 664–674, 2016.

[340] Terence C Mills. *Applied Time Series Analysis: A Practical Guide to Modeling and Forecasting*. Academic Press, 2019.

[341] Brenda Milner. Effects of different brain lesions on card sorting: The role of the frontal lobes. *Archives of Neurology*, 9(1): 90–100, 1963.

[342] Gabriel T Mindler, Andreas Kranzl, Alexandra Stauffer, Gabriele Haeusler, Rudolf Ganger et al. Disease-specific gait deviations in pediatric patients with x-linked hypophosphatemia. *Gait & Posture*, 81: 78–84, 2020.

[343] Goverdhan Mogli. Role of biometrics in healthcare privacy and security management system. *Sri Lanka Journal of Bio-Medical Informatics*, 2(4), 2012.

[344] Zeynab Mohammadi, Javad Frounchi and Mahmood Amiri. Wavelet-based emotion recognition system using eeg signal. *Neural Computing and Applications*, 28(8): 1985–1990, 2017.

[345] M Mohammed, B Abdelmadjid and B Djamila. A fuzzy logic controller for electric powered wheelchair based on lagrange model. In *2019 International Conference on Advanced Electrical Engineering (ICAEE)*, pp. 1–6, 2019.

[346] AH Mohsin, AA Zaidan, BB Zaidan, OS Albahri, Shamsul Arrieya Bin Ariffin et al. Finger vein biometrics: Taxonomy analysis, open challenges, future directions, and recommended solution for decentralised network architectures. *IEEE Access*, 8: 9821–9845, 2020.

[347] Jeffrey Montes, John Young, Richard Tandy and James Navalta. Fitbit flex: Energy expenditure and step count evaluation. *Journal of Exercise Physiology Online*, 20: 152–158, 10 2017.

[348] Keith Morgan. The benefits of in-home, monitored eeg testing. Available at https://www.beckershospitalreview.com/healthcare-informationtechnology/the-benefits-of-in-home-monitored-eeg-testing.html (accessed: 2021-05-11), September 2017.

[349] Donald E Morisky, Lawrence W Green and David M Levine. Concurrent and predictive validity of a self-reported measure of medication adherence. *Medical Care*, 67–74, 1986.

[350] Andrew Morley and Lizzie Hill. 10–20 system EEG Placement. Available at www.ers-education.org/lrmedia/2016/pdf/298830.pdf (accessed: 2021-05-11), 2013.

[351] Frank Morrell, Lamar Roberts and Herbert H Jasper. Effect of focal epileptogenic lesions and their ablation upon conditioned electrical responses of the brain in the monkey. *Electroencephalography and Clinical Neurophysiology*, 8(2): 217–236, 1956.

[352] HK Mukhopadhyay, Sanjay Kumar Das, Lakshmikanta Ghosh and Bijan Kumar Gupta. Epilepsy and its management: A review. *Journal of PharmaSciTech*, 1(2): 20–26, 2012.

[353] Thangaraj Munusamy, Ravindran Karuppiah, Nor Faizal A Bahuri, Sutharshan Sockalingam, Chun Yoong Cham et al. Telemedicine via smart glasses in critical care of the neurosurgical patient—covid-19 pandemic preparedness and response in neurosurgery. *World Neurosurgery*, 145: e53–e60, 2021.

[354] Juana Isabel Méndez, Omar Mata, Pedro Ponce, Alan Meier, Therese Peffer et al. Multi-sensor system, gamification, and artificial intelligence for benefit elderly people. pp. 207–235. *In*: Hiram Ponce, Lourdes Martínez-Villaseñor, Jorge Brieva and Ernesto Moya-Albor (eds.). *Challenges and Trends in Multimodal Fall Detection for Healthcare*, volume 273. Springer International Publishing, Cham, 2020.

[355] NI Katevas, NM Sgouros, SG Tzafestas, G Papakonstantinou, P Beattie et al. The autonomous mobile robot SENARIO: A sensor aided intelligent navigation system for powered wheelchairs. *IEEE Robotics & Automation Magazine*, 4(4): 60–70, December 1997.

[356] Sugan Nagarajan, Satya Sai Srinivas Nettimi, Lakshmi Sutha Kumar, Malaya Kumar Nath and Aniruddha Kanhe. Speech emotion recognition using cepstral features extracted with novel triangular filter banks based on bark and erb frequency scales. *Digital Signal Processing*, 104: 102763, 2020.

[357] Takashi Nakamura, Valentin Goverdovsky and Danilo P Mandic. In-ear eeg biometrics for feasible and readily collectable real-world person authentication. *IEEE Transactions on Information Forensics and Security*, 13(3): 648–661, 2018.

[358] Ilya Naplekov, Ivan Zheleznikov, Dmitry Pashchenko, Polina Kobysheva, Anna Moskvitina et al. Methods of computational modeling of coronary heart vessels for its digital twin. *MATEC Web of Conferences*, 172: 1–6, 2018.

[359] Mihir Narayan Mohanty and Rishi Sikka. Review on fingerprint-based identification system. *Materials Today: Proceedings*, 2021.

[360] Marta Nave, Paulo Rita and João Guerreiro. A decision support system framework to track consumer sentiments in social media. *Journal of Hospitality Marketing & Management*, 27(6): 693–710, 2018.

[361] Bernd A Neubauer and Andreas Hahn. *Dooses Epilepsien im Kindes-und Jugendalter*, volume 12. Springer, 2012.

[362] Daniel Nguyen, Jean Jeudy, Alejandro Jimenez Restrepo and Timm-Michael Dickfeld. A novel use of noninvasive registered electrocardiographic imaging map for localization of vt and pvc. *JACC: Case Reports*, 3(4): 591–593, 2021.

[363] Nicoletta Nicolaou and Julius Georgiou. Detection of epileptic electroencephalogram based on permutation entropy and support vector machines. *Expert Systems with Applications*, 39(1): 202–209, 2012.

[364] Antonio Gennaro Nicotera, Randi Jenssen Hagerman, Maria Vincenza Catania, Serafino Buono, Santo Di Nuovo et al. Eeg abnormalities as a neurophysiological biomarker of severity in autism spectrum disorder: A pilot cohort study. *Journal of Autism and Developmental Disorders*, 49(6):2337–2347, 2019.

[365] S Noachtar, C Binnie, J Ebersole, F Mauguiere, A Sakamoto et al. A glossary of terms most commonly used by clinical electroencephalographers and proposal for the report form for the EEG findings the international federation of Clinical Neurophysiology. *Electroencephalography and Clinical Neurophysiology. Supplement*, 52: 21, 1999.

[366] S Noachtar, H Holthausen, A Sakamoto, H Pannek and P Wolf. Semi-invasive elektroden in der epilepsiechirurgischen diagnostik. *Epilepsie*, 92: 148–52, 1993.

[367] Soheyl Noachtar and Jan Rémi. The role of EEG in epilepsy: A critical review. *Epilepsy & Behavior*, 15(1): 22–33, 2009.

[368] William S Noble. What is a support vector machine? *Nature Biotechnology*, 24(12): 1565–1567, 2006.

[369] Jakub Novotný. Sport wearables from the first heart rate monitor to online services. In *Proceedings of the 24rd International Conference on System approaches 2018. System Perspective on Modern Media*, p. 13, 2018.

[370] Amin Nozariasbmarz, Henry Collins, Kelvin Dsouza, Mobarak Hossain Polash, Mahshid Hosseini et al. Review of wearable thermoelectric energy harvesting: From body temperature to electronic systems. *Applied Energy*, 258: 114069, 2020.

[371] Nahumi Nugrahaningsih and Marco Porta. Soft biometrics through hand gestures driven by visual stimuli. *ICT Express*, 5(2): 94–99, 2019.

[372] Mohammad S Obaidat, Soumya Prakash Rana, Tanmoy Maitra, Debasis Giri and Subrata Dutta. *Biometric Security and Internet of Things (IOT)*. Springer, 2018.

[373] University of Bonn. D. of epileptology. http://www.meb.unibonn.de/epileptologie/science/physik/eegdata.html (accessed: 2021-05-11), 2021.

[374] Obi Ogbanufe and Dan J Kim. Comparing fingerprint-based biometrics authentication versus traditional authentication methods for e-payment. *Decision Support Systems*, 106: 1–14, 2018.

[375] Oliveira Johnatan, Souza Gustavo, Rocha Anderson, Deus Flavio and Marana Aparecido. Cross-domain deep face matching for real banking security systems. Available online (accessed: 2021-05-11), 2018.

[376] Muhtahir O Oloyede and Gerhard P Hancke. Unimodal and multimodal biometric sensing systems: A review. *IEEE Access*, 4: 7532–7555, 2016.

[377] Robert Oostenveld, Pascal Fries, Eric Maris and Jan-Mathijs Schoffelen. Fieldtrip: Open source software for advanced analysis of meg, eeg, and invasive electrophysiological data. *Computational Intelligence and Neuroscience*, 2011, 2011.

[378] Orrin Devinsky, Epilepsy Foundation. Video-EEG Monitoring. Available at https://www.epilepsy.com/living-epilepsy/epilepsy-and/professional-healthcare-providers/about-epilepsy-seizures/classifying-seizures/nonepilepticseizures/diagnosis/video-eeg-monitoring (accessed: 2021-05-11), 2004.

[379] Rupert Ortner, Engelbert Grünbacher and Christoph Guger. State of the art in sensors, signals and signal processing. *Gtecjapan. Com*, pp. 1–18, 2013.

[380] Ivan Osorio, Mary Ann F Harrison, Ying-Cheng Lai and Mark G Frei. Observations on the application of the correlation dimension and correlation integral to the prediction of seizures. *Journal of Clinical Neurophysiology*, 18(3): 269–274, 2001.

[381] R Ouch, B Garcia-Zapirain and R Yampolskiy. Multimodal biometrie systems: A systematic review. In *2017 IEEE International Symposium on Signal Processing and Information Technology (ISSPIT)*, pp. 439–444, Dec 2017.

[382] Emmanuel Kwame Owusu-Oware, John Effah and Richard Boateng. Biometric technology for fighting fraud in national health insurance: Ghana's experience. In *24th Americas Conference on Information Systems, AMCIS 2018, New Orleans, LA, USA, August 16–18, 2018*. Association for Information Systems, 2018.

[383] Alison M Pack. Epilepsy overview and revised classification of seizures and epilepsies. *Continuum: Lifelong Learning in Neurology*, 25(2): 306–321, 2019.

[384] Edward B Panganiban, Arnold C Paglinawan, Wen Yaw Chung and Gilbert Lance S Paa. Ecg diagnostic support system (edss): A deep learning neural network based classification system for detecting ecg abnormal rhythms from a low-powered wearable biosensors. *Sensing and Bio-Sensing Research*, 31: 100398, 2021.

[385] Sharath Pankanti, Ruud M Bolle and Anil Jain. Biometrics: The future of identification [guest editors' introduction]. *Computer*, 33(2): 46–49, 2000.

[386] Gabriella Panuccio, Marianna Semprini, Lorenzo Natale, Stefano Buccelli, Ilaria Colombi et al. Progress in neuroengineering for brain repair: New challenges and open issues. *Brain and Neuroscience Advances*, 2: 2398212818776475, 2018.

[387] Harsh Panwar, PK Gupta, Mohammad Khubeb Siddiqui, Ruben Morales-Menendez and Vaishnavi Singh. Application of deep learning for fast detection of covid-19 in x-rays using ncovnet. *Chaos, Solitons & Fractals*, 109944, 2020.

[388] Sajeesh Parameswaran, Anu Mohan et al. Acute electrocorticography (ecog) during mesial temporal lobe epilepsy surgery-review. *Open Access Journal of Neurology & Neurosurgery*, 7(5): 95–98, 2018.

[389] Bens Pardamean, Haryono Soeparno, Arif Budiarto, Bharuno Mahesworo and James Baurley. Quantified self-using consumer wearable device: Predicting physical and mental health. *Healthcare Informatics Research*, 26(2): 83–92, Apr 2020.

[390] Bens Pardamean, Haryono Soeparno, Bharuno Mahesworo, Arif Budiarto and James Baurley. Comparing the accuracy of multiple commercial wearable devices: A method. *Procedia Computer Science*, 157: 567–572, 2019. The 4th International Conference on Computer Science and Computational Intelligence (ICCSCI 2019): Enabling Collaboration to Escalate Impact of Research Results for Society.

[391] Kellow Pardini, Joel JPC Rodrigues, Ousmane Diallo, Ashok Kumar Das, Victor Hugo C de Albuquerque et al. A smart waste management solution geared towards citizens. *Sensors (Switzerland)*, 20(8): 1–15, 2020.

[392] Joseph Pato and Lynnette Millett. *Biometric Recognition: Challenges and Opportunities*. National Research Council, 2010.

[393] Raymond Pearl et al. *Introduction to Medical Biometry and Statistics*. London: WB Saunders Company, 1930.

[394] Luiz Pessoa. Understanding brain networks and brain organization. *Physics of Life Reviews*, 11(3): 400–435, 2014.

[395] Vladimir S Petrović and Costas S Xydeas. Sensor noise effects on signal-level image fusion performance. *Information Fusion*, 4(3): 167–183, 2003.

[396] A Pflug and C Busch. Ear biometrics: A survey of detection, feature extraction and recognition methods. *IET Biometrics*, 1(2): 114–129, June 2012.

[397] Angkoon Phinyomark, Pornchai Phukpattaranont and Chusak Limsakul. A review of control methods for electric power wheelchairs based on electromyography signals with special emphasis on pattern recognition. *IETE Technical Review*, 28(4): 316–326, July 2011. Publisher: Taylor & Francis.

[398] Steven M Pincus. Approximate entropy as a measure of system complexity. *Proceedings of the National Academy of Sciences*, 88(6): 2297–2301, 1991.

[399] Luca Pion-Tonachini, Ken Kreutz-Delgado and Scott Makeig. Iclabel: An automated electroencephalographic independent component classifier, dataset, and website. *NeuroImage*, 198: 181–197, 2019.

[400] Sandeep Pirbhulal, Heye Zhang, Subhas Chandra Mukhopadhyay, Chunyue Li, Yumei Wang et al. An efficient biometric-based algorithm using heart rate variability for securing body sensor networks. *Sensors*, 15(7): 15067–15089, 2015.

[401] G Pires, U Nunes and AT de Almeida. RobChair—A semi-autonomous wheelchair for disabled people. *3rd IFAC Symposium on Intelligent Autonomous Vehicles 1998 (IAV'98), Madrid, Spain, 25–27 March*, 31(3): 509–513, March 1998.

[402] Gabriel Pires and Urbano Nunes. A wheelchair steered through voice commands and assisted by a reactive fuzzy-logic controller. *Journal of Intelligent and Robotic Systems*, 34(3): 301–314, July 2002.

[403] Malgorzata Plechawska-Wojcik, Monika Kaczorowska and Dariusz Zapala. The artifact subspace reconstruction (asr) for eeg signal correction. a comparative study. In *International Conference on Information Systems Architecture and Technology*, pp. 125–135. Springer, 2018.

[404] Ming-Zher Poh, Tobias Loddenkemper, Nicholas C Swenson, Shubhi Goyal, Joseph R Madsen et al. Continuous monitoring of electrodermal activity during epileptic seizures using a wearable sensor. In *2010 Annual International Conference of the IEEE Engineering in Medicine and Biology*, pp. 4415–4418. IEEE, 2010.

[405] Pedro Ponce, Arturo Molina, Rafael Mendoza, Marco Antonio Ruiz, David Gregory Monnard et al. Intelligent wheelchair and virtual training by LabVIEW. pp. 422–435. *In*: Grigori Sidorov, Arturo Hernández Aguirre and Carlos Alberto Reyes García (eds.). Advances in Artificial Intelligence, Berlin, Heidelberg, 2010. Springer Berlin Heidelberg.

[406] Pedro Ponce Cruz and Fernando D Ramírez-Figueroa. *Intelligent Control Systems with LabVIEW*. Springer, London; New York, 2010. OCLC: ocn506258307.

[407] Marco Porta and Alessandro Barboni. Strengthening security in industrial settings: A study on gaze-based biometrics through free observation of static images. In *2019 24th IEEE International Conference on Emerging Technologies and Factory Automation (ETFA)*, pp. 1273–1277, 2019.

[408] Carolina Graña Possamai, Philippe Ravaud, Lina Ghosn and Viet-Thi Tran. Use of wearable biometric monitoring devices to measure outcomes in randomized clinical trials: A methodological systematic review. *BMC Medicine*, 18(1): 1–11, 2020.

[409] Sara Pourmohammadi and Ali Maleki. Stress detection using ecg and emg signals: A comprehensive study. *Computer Methods and Programs in Biomedicine*, 193: 105482, 2020.

[410] David MW Powers. Evaluation: from precision, recall and f-measure to roc, informedness, markedness and correlation. *arXiv preprint arXiv:2010.16061*, 2020.

[411] Salil Prabhakar, Alexander Ivanisov and Anil Jain. Biometric recognition: Sensor characteristics and image quality. *IEEE Instrumentation & Mmeasurement Magazine*, 14(3): 10–16, 2011.

[412] Olga Prilipko, Jacqueline Delavelle, Francois Lazeyras and Margitta Seeck. Reversible cytotoxic edema in the splenium of the corpus callosum related to antiepileptic treatment: report of two cases and literature review. *Epilepsia*, 46(10): 1633–1636, 2005.

[413] Dilok Puanhvuan, Sarawin Khemmachotikun, Pongsakorn Wechakarn, Boonyanuch Wijarn and Yodchanan Wongsawat. Navigation-synchronized multimodal control wheelchair from brain to alternative assistive technologies for persons with severe disabilities. *Cognitive Neurodynamics*, 11(2): 117–134, April 2017.

[414] J Ross Quinlan. Induction of decision trees. *Machine Learning*, 1(1): 81–106, 1986.

[415] RC Simpson, D Poirot and F Baxter. The Hephaestus smart wheelchair system. *IEEE Transactions on Neural Systems and Rehabilitation Engineering*, 10(2): 118–122, June 2002.

[416] RC Simpson and SP Levine. Voice control of a powered wheelchair. *IEEE Transactions on Neural Systems and Rehabilitation Engineering*, 10(2): 122–125, June 2002.

[417] R Madarasz, L Heiny, R Cromp and N Mazur. The design of an autonomous vehicle for the disabled. *IEEE Journal on Robotics and Automation*, 2(3): 117–126, September 1986.

[418] RS Soundariya and R Renuga. Eye movement based emotion recognition using electrooculography. In *2017 Innovations in Power and Advanced Computing Technologies (i-PACT)*, pp. 1–5, April 2017. Journal Abbreviation: 2017 Innovations in Power and Advanced Computing Technologies (i-PACT).

[419] Yassine Rabhi, Makrem Mrabet and Farhat Fnaiech. A facial expression controlled wheelchair for people with disabilities. *Computer Methods and Programs in Biomedicine*, 165: 89–105, October 2018.

[420] Thea Radüntz and Beate Meffert. Cross-modality matching for evaluating user experience of emerging mobile eeg technology. *IEEE Transactions on Human-Machine Systems*, 50(4): 298–305, 2020.

[421] R Raghavendra and Christoph Busch. A low cost wrist vein sensor for biometric authentication. In *Imaging Systems and Techniques (IST), 2016 IEEE International Conference on*, pp. 201–205. IEEE, 2016.

[422] R Raghavendra, Jayachander Surbiryala and Christoph Busch. Hand dorsal vein recognition: Sensor, algorithms and evaluation. In *2015 IEEE International Conference on Imaging Systems and Techniques (IST)*, pp. 1–6. IEEE, 2015.

[423] Bhargavi Ramanujam, Deepa Dash and Manjari Tripathi. Can home videos made on smartphones complement video-eeg in diagnosing psychogenic nonepileptic seizures? *Seizure*, 62: 95–98, 2018.

[424] Thomas Z Ramsøy, Catrine Jacobsen, Morten Friis-Olivarius, Dalia Bagdziunaite and Martin Skov. Predictive value of body posture and pupil dilation in assessing consumer preference and choice. *Journal of Neuroscience Psychology and Economics*, 08 2017.

[425] Nalini Kanta Ratha and Venu Govindaraju. *Advances in Biometrics: Sensors, Algorithms and Systems*. Springer Science & Business Media, 2007.

[426] D Rating. Journal club, wie konstant ist die eeg-befundung? *Zeitschrift fuer Epileptologie*, 27(2): 139–142, 2014.

[427] Vipula Rawte and G Anuradha. Fraud detection in health insurance using data mining techniques. In *2015 International Conference on Communication, Information & Computing Technology (ICCICT)*, pp. 1–5. IEEE, 2015.

[428] Philipp S Reif, Adam Strzelczyk and Felix Rosenow. The history of invasive EEG evaluation in epilepsy patients. *Seizure*, 41: 191–195, 2016.

[429] JD Reiss. *The Analysis of Chaotic Time Series*. PhD thesis, Georgia Institute of Technology, 2001.

[430] Chun-xiao Ren, Yu-bin Gong, Fei Hao, Xin-yan Cai and Yu-xiao Wu. When biometrics meet iot: A survey. pp. 635–643. *In*: Ershi Qi (ed.). *Proceedings of the 6th International Asia Conference on Industrial Engineering and Management Innovation*, Paris, 2016. Atlantis Press.

[431] Edward H Reynolds, NE Bharucha and JW Sander. Epilepsy: The disorder. *Epilepst Atlas*, WHO, pp. 16–27, 2005.

[432] Edward H Reynolds and James V Kinnier Wilson. Psychoses of epilepsy in babylon: The oldest account of the disorder. *Epilepsia*, 49(9): 1488–1490, 2008.

[433] Joshua S Richman and J Randall Moorman. Physiological time-series analysis using approximate entropy and sample entropy. *American Journal of Physiology-Heart and Circulatory Physiology*, 278(6): H2039–H2049, 2000.

[434] Roberto Roizenblatt, Paulo Schor, Fabio Dante, Jaime Roizenblatt and Rubens Jr Belfort. Iris recognition as a biometric method after cataract surgery. *Biomedical Engineering Online*, 3: 2, Jan 2004.

[435] Mario Rojas, Pedro Ponce and Arturo Molina. Skills based evaluation of alternative input methods to command a semi-autonomous electric wheelchair. *Conference proceedings: ... Annual International Conference of the IEEE Engineering in Medicine and Biology Society. IEEE Engineering in Medicine and Biology Society. Annual Conference*, 2016: 4593–4596, August 2016. Place: United States.

[436] Mario Rojas, Pedro Ponce and Arturo Molina. A fuzzy logic navigation controller implemented in hardware for an electric wheelchair. *International Journal of Advanced Robotic Systems*, 15(1): 1729881418755768, January 2018. Publisher: SAGE Publications.

[437] Jeremy Rose. Biometrics as a service: The next giant leap? *Biometric Technology Today*, 2016(3): 7–9, 2016.

[438] Michael T Rosenstein, James J Collins and Carlo J De Luca. A practical method for calculating largest lyapunov exponents from small data sets. *Physica D: Nonlinear Phenomena*, 65(1-2): 117–134, 1993.

[439] Arun Ross, Sudipta Banerjee, Cunjian Chen, Anurag Chowdhury, Vahid Mirjalili et al. Some research problems in biometrics: The future beckons. In *2019 International Conference on Biometrics (ICB)*, pp. 1–8. IEEE, 2019.

[440] Ryan M Rothschild. Neuroengineering tools/applications for bidirectional interfaces, brain–computer interfaces, and neuroprosthetic implants–a review of recent progress. *Frontiers in Neuroengineering*, 3: 112, 2010.

[441] Lourdes Cecilia RUIZ and Tibor KOVACS. Biometric screenings: The route to occupational safety and health. *Journal of Scientific Perspectives*, 5(1): 25–35, 2021.

[442] Artur Rygula. Driving style identification method based on speed graph analysis. In *2009 International Conference on Biometrics and Kansei Engineering*, pp. 76–79. IEEE, 2009.

[443] S Desai, SS Mantha and VM Phalle. Advances in smart wheelchair technology. In *2017 International Conference on Nascent Technologies in Engineering (ICNTE)*, pp. 1–7, January 2017. Journal Abbreviation: 2017 International Conference on Nascent Technologies in Engineering (ICNTE).

[444] ME Saab and Jean Gotman. A system to detect the onset of epileptic seizures in scalp EEG. *Clinical Neurophysiology*, 116(2): 427–442, 2005.

[445] T Sabhanayagam, V Prasanna Venkatesan and K Senthamaraikannan. A comprehensive survey on various biometric systems. International Journal of Applied Engineering Research, 13(5): 2276–2297, 2018.

[446] Hanan Samet. K-nearest neighbor finding using maxnearestdist. *IEEE Transactions on Pattern Analysis and Machine Intelligence*, 30(2): 243–252, 2007.

[447] Øyvind Sandbakk. The role of sport science in the new age of digital sport. *International Journal of Sports Physiology and Performance*, 15(2): 153, 2020.

[448] Rene Santos, Jorge Oliveira, Jessica Rocha and Janaina Giraldi. Eye tracking in neuromarketing: A research agenda for marketing studies. *International Journal of Psychological Studies*, 7, 02 2015.

[449] Sergio Saponara. Biometric performance measurements in combat sports. In *2016 IEEE International Symposium on Medical Measurements and Applications (MeMeA)*, pp. 1–5, 2016.

[450] Shahenda Sarhan, Shaaban Alhassan and Samir Elmougy. Multimodal biometric systems: A comparative study. *Arabian Journal for Science and Engineering*, 42(2): 443–457, 2017.

[451] Iqbal H Sarker, Hamed Alqahtani, Fawaz Alsolami, Asif Irshad Khan, Yoosef B Abushark et al. Context premodeling: An empirical analysis for classification based user-centric context aware predictive modeling. *Journal of Big Data*, 7(1): 1–23, 2020.

[452] Steven C Schachter, PO Shafer and JI Sirven. What causes epilepsy and seizures. *Epilepsy Foundation*, 2013.

[453] Mark C Jr Schall, Richard F Sesek and Lora A Cavuoto. Barriers to the adoption of wearable sensors in the workplace: A survey of occupational safety and health professionals. *Human Factors*, 60(3): 351–362, May 2018.

[454] Ingrid E Scheffer, Samuel Berkovic, Giuseppe Capovilla, Mary B Connolly, Jacqueline French et al. Ilae classification of the epilepsies: Position paper of the ilae commission for classification and terminology. *Epilepsia*, 58(4): 512–521, 2017.

[455] MScher. Neonatal seizures: An expression of fetal or neonatal brain disorders. *Fetal and Neonatal Brain Injury. Mechanisms, Management and the Risks of Practice*, pp. 735–784, 2003.

[456] Bernhard Schmitt and Gabriele Wohlrab. Eeg in der neuropädiatrie. In *Klinische Elektroenzephalographie*, pp. 523–585. Springer, 2012.

[457] M Schukat, D McCaldin, K Wang, G Schreier, N Lovell et al. Unintended consequences of wearable sensor use in healthcare contribution of the imia wearable sensors in healthcare wg. *Yearbook of Medical Informatics*, 1: 73–86, 2016.

[458] Steven M Schwartz, Kevin Wildenhaus, Amy Bucher and Brigid Byrd. Digital twins and the emerging science of self: Implications for digital health experience design and "small" data. *Frontiers in Computer Science*, 2(October): 1–16, 2020.

[459] Seattle Children's, Seattle, Washington. Ambulatory EEG monitoring. What to expect from EEG monitoring at home. Available at https://www. seattlechildrens.org/globalassets/documents/for-patients-andfamilies/pfe/ pe1379.pdf (accessed: 2021-05-11), 2019.

[460] Adrien Sedeaud, Andy Marc, Julien Schipman, Karine Schaal, Mario Danial et al. Secular trend: Morphology and performance. *Journal of Sports Sciences*, 32(12): 1146–1154, 2014.

[461] D Selvathi and Henry Selvaraj. Fpga implementation for epileptic seizure detection using amplitude and frequency analysis of eeg signals. In *2017 25th International Conference on Systems Engineering (ICSEng)*, pp. 183–192. IEEE, 2017.

[462] Carlo Semenza. Impairment in localization of body parts following brain damage. *Cortex*, 24(3): 443–449, 1988.

[463] Sudhakar Sengan, Kailash Kumar, V Subramaniyaswamy and Logesh Ravi. Cost-effective and efficient 3D human model creation and re-

identification application for human digital twins. *Multimedia Tools and Applications*, 2021.

[464] Mohsin Shafiq, Imtiaz A Taj, Mubeen Ghafoor, Syed Ali Tariq, Assad Abbas et al. Accelerating fingerprint identification using fpga for large-scale applications. *Journal of Parallel and Distributed Computing*, 141: 35–48, 2020.

[465] Dhvani Shah and Vinayak haradi. Iot based biometrics implementation on raspberry pi. *Procedia Computer Science*, 79: 328–336, 2016. Proceedings of International Conference on Communication, Computing and Virtualization (ICCCV) 2016.

[466] Claude Elwood Shannon. A mathematical theory of communication. *The Bell System Technical Journal*, 27(3): 379–423, 1948.

[467] Frank Sharbrough. American electroencephalographic society guidelines for standard electrode position nomenclature. *J Clin Neurophysiol*, 8: 200–202, 1991.

[468] Shilpa Sharma and Kumud Sachdeva. Face recognition using pca and svm with surf technique. *International Journal of Computer Applications*, 129: 41–46, 11 2015.

[469] Tsu-Wang Shen, Xavier Kuo and Yue-Loong Hsin. Ant k-means clustering method on epileptic spike detection. In *2009 Fifth International Conference on Natural Computation*, volume 6, pages 334–338. IEEE, 2009.

[470] Xu Shen, Ibukun Awolusi and Eric Marks. Construction equipment operator physiological data assessment and tracking. *Practice Periodical on Structural Design and Construction*, 22(4): 04017006, 2017.

[471] Matthew Shere, Hansung Kim and Adrian Hilton. 3d human pose estimation from multi person stereo 360 scenes. In *Proceedings of the IEEE/CVF Conference on Computer Vision and Pattern Recognition (CVPR) Workshops*, June 2019.

[472] Ming-Yuan Shieh, Juing-Shian Chiou, Yu-Chia Hu and Kuo-YangWang. Applications of pca and svm-pso based real-time face recognition system. *Mathematical Problems in Engineering*, 2014: 1–12, 05 2014.

[473] Kyong Jin Shin, Jong Woo Kang, Kwon Hyuk Sung, Sung Ho Park, Si Eun Kim et al. Quantitative gait and postural analyses in patients with diabetic polyneuropathy. *Journal of Diabetes and its Complications*, 35(4): 107857, 2021.

[474] Ali H Shoeb and John V Guttag. Application of machine learning to epileptic seizure detection. In *Proceedings of the 27th International Conference on Machine Learning (ICML-10)*, pp. 975–982, 2010.

[475] Simon Shorvon and Torbjorn Tomson. Sudden unexpected death in epilepsy. *The Lancet*, 378(9808): 2028–2038, 2011.

[476] Mohammad Khubeb Siddiqui. *Brain Data Mining for Epileptic Seizure Detection*. PhD thesis, Doctoral Thesis, Charles Sturt University, Australia, 2018.

[477] Mohammad Khubeb Siddiqui, Xiaodi Huang, Ruben Morales-Menendez, Nasir Hussain and Khudeja Khatoon. Machine learning based novel costsensitive seizure detection classifier for imbalanced eeg data sets. *International Journal on Interactive Design and Manufacturing*, 14: 1491–1509, October 2020.

[478] Mohammad Khubeb Siddiqui and Md Zahidul Islam. Data mining approach in seizure detection. In *2016 IEEE Region 10 Conference (TENCON)*, pp. 3579–3583. IEEE, 2016.

[479] Mohammad Khubeb Siddiqui, Md Zahidul Islam and Muhammad Ashad Kabir. Analyzing performance of classification techniques in detecting epileptic seizure. In *International Conference on Advanced Data Mining and Applications*, pp. 386–398. Springer, 2017.

[480] Mohammad Khubeb Siddiqui, Md Zahidul Islam and Muhammad Ashad Kabir. A novel quick seizure detection and localization through brain data mining on ECoG dataset. *Neural Computing and Applications*, 31(9): 5595–5608, 2019.

[481] Mohammad Khubeb Siddiqui, Ruben Morales-Menendez and Sultan Ahmad. Application of receiver operating characteristics (roc) on the prediction of obesity. *Brazilian Archives of Biology and Technology*, 63, 2020.

[482] Mohammad Khubeb Siddiqui, Ruben Morales-Menendez, Pradeep Kumar Gupta, HM Iqbal, Fida Hussain et al. Correlation between temperature and covid-19 (suspected, confirmed and death) cases based on machine learning analysis. *J Pure Appl Microbiol*, 14, 2020.

[483] Mohammad Khubeb Siddiqui, Ruben Morales-Menendez, Xiaodi Huang and Nasir Hussain. A review of epileptic seizure detection using machine learning classifiers. *Brain Informatics*, 7(1): 1–18, 2020.

[484] Mohammad Khubeb Siddiqui and Shams Naahid. Analysis of kdd cup 99 dataset using clustering based data mining. *International Journal of Database Theory and Application*, 6(5): 23–34, 2013.

[485] David Christopher Balderas Silva, Pedro Ponce Cruz, Arturo Molina Gutiérrez and Luis Arturo Soriano Avendaño. *Applications of Human-Computer Interaction and Robotics based on Artificial Intelligence.* Editorial Digital del Tecnológico de Monterrey, January 2020.

[486] Richard Simpson, Edmund Lopresti, Steve Hayashi, Illah Nourbakhsh and David Miller. The smart wheelchair component system. *Journal of Rehabilitation Research and Development*, 41(3B): 429–442, May 2004. Place: United States.

[487] G Sintotskiy and H Hinrichs. In-ear-eeg–a portable platform for home monitoring. *Journal of Medical Engineering & Technology*, 44(1): 26–37, 2020.

[488] Joseph I Sirven. Electrocorticogram (ecog). In *Encyclopedia of the Neurological Sciences*, pp. 1080–1083. Elsevier Inc., 2014.

[489] Andrew L Skinner, Christopher J Stone, Hazel Doughty and Marcus R Munafò. Stopwatch: The preliminary evaluation of a smartwatch-based system for passive detection of cigarette smoking. *Nicotine and Tobacco Research*, 21(2): 257–261, 2019.

[490] Matt Smallman. Why voice is getting stronger in financial services. *Biometric Technology Today*, 2017(1): 5–7, 2017.

[491] Stephen M Smith. Fast robust automated brain extraction. *Human Brain Mapping*, 17(3): 143–155, 2002.

[492] Robert R Sokal. Biometry: The Principles and Practice of Statistics. *Biological Research*, 1995.

[493] Sharon Eve Sonenblum, Stephen Sprigle, Jayme Caspall and Ricardo Lopez. Validation of an accelerometer-based method to measure the use of manual wheelchairs. *Medical Engineering & Physics*, 34(6): 781–786, July 2012.

[494] Julien Clinton Sprott. *Chaos and Time-series Analysis*, volume 69. Citeseer, 2003.

[495] Carl E Stafstrom and Lionel Carmant. Seizures and epilepsy: An overview for neuroscientists. *Cold Spring Harbor Perspectives in Medicine*, 5(6): a022426, 2015.

[496] Kevin J Staley, Andrew White and F Edward Dudek. Interictal spikes: Harbingers or causes of epilepsy? *Neuroscience Letters*, 497(3): 247–250, 2011.

[497] Cornelis Jan Stam. Chaos, continuous eeg, and cognitive mechanisms: A future for clinical neurophysiology. *American Journal of Electroneurodiagnostic Technology*, 43(4): 211–227, 2003.

[498] Vince Stanford. Biosignals offer potential for direct interfaces and health monitoring. *IEEE Pervasive Computing*, 3(1): 99–103, 2004.

[499] Thanos G Stavropoulos, Asterios Papastergiou, Lampros Mpaltadoros, Spiros Nikolopoulos and Ioannis Kompatsiaris. Iot wearable sensors and devices in elderly care: A literature review. *Sensors*, 20(10): 2826, 2020.

[500] Elena Stefana, Filippo Marciano, Diana Rossi, Paola Cocca and Giuseppe Tomasoni. Wearable devices for ergonomics: A systematic literature review. *Sensors (Basel, Switzerland)*, 21(3), Jan 2021.

[501] Ulrich Stephani. The natural history of myoclonic astatic epilepsy (doose syndrome) and lennox-gastaut syndrome. *Epilepsia*, 47: 53–55, 2006.

[502] Arkadiusz Stopczynski, Carsten Stahlhut, Michael Kai Petersen, Jakob Eg Larsen, Camilla Falk Jensen et al. Smartphones as pocketable labs: Visions for mobile brain imaging and neurofeedback. *International Journal of Psychophysiology*, 91(1): 54–66, 2014.

[503] Andrew T Stull, Logan Fiorella and Richard E Mayer. An eye-tracking analysis of instructor presence in video lectures. *Computers in Human Behavior*, 88: 263–272, 2018.

[504] Ioannis Stylios, Spyros Kokolakis, Olga Thanou and Sotirios Chatzis. Behavioral biometrics and continuous user authentication on mobile devices: A survey. *Information Fusion*, 66: 76–99, 2021.

[505] Vladimir N Sudakov. *Geometric Problems in the Theory of Infinite-Dimensional Probability Distributions*, volume 141. American Mathematical Soc., 1979.

[506] Madeena Sultana, Padma Polash Paul and Marina Gavrilova. A concept of social behavioral biometrics: Motivation, current developments, and future trends. *Proceedings—2014 International Conference on Cyberworlds, CW 2014*, pp. 271–278, 2014.

[507] Madeena Sultana, Padma Polash Paul and Marina L Gavrilova. User recognition from social behavior in computer-mediated social context. *IEEE Transactions on Human-Machine Systems*, 47(3): 356–367, 2017.

[508] Jianshan Sun, Zhiqiang Tian, Yelin Fu, Jie Geng and Chunli Liu. Digital twins in human understanding: A deep learning-based method to recognize personality traits. *International Journal of Computer Integrated Manufacturing*, 00(00): 1–14, 2020.

[509] Kenji Suzuki. Artificial neural networks: Architectures and applications. *IntechOpen*, 2013.

[510] Jerzy Szulga. *Introduction to Random Chaos*. CRC Press, 1998.

[511] Juri Taborri, Justin Keogh, Anton Kos, Alessandro Santuz, Anton Umek et al. Sport biomechanics applications using inertial, force, and emg sensors: A literature overview. Applied Bionics and Biomechanics, 2020: 2041549, 2020.

[512] H Takao, N Hayashi and K Ohtomo. Brain diffusivity pattern is individual specific information. *Neuroscience*, 301: 395–402, 2015.

[513] Ripple Talati, Jennifer M Scholle, Olivia J Phung, William L Baker, Erica L Baker et al. Effectiveness and safety of antiepileptic medications in patients with epilepsy. Agency for Healthcare Research and Quality (US), 2012.

[514] Michelle Taub and Roger Azevedo. How does prior knowledge influence eye fixations and sequences of cognitive and metacognitive srl processes during learning with an intelligent tutoring system? *International Journal of Artificial Intelligence in Education*, 29(1): 1–28, Mar 2019.

[515] Henrique Leal Tavares, João Baptista Cardia Neto, João Paulo Papa, Danilo Colombo and Aparecido Nilceu Marana. Tracking and re-identification of people using soft-biometrics. In *2019 XV Workshop de Visão Computacional (WVC)*, pp. 78–83, 2019.

[516] Nattapong Thammasan, Ivo V Stuldreher, Elisabeth Schreuders, Matteo Giletta and Anne-Marie Brouwer. A usability study of physiological measurement in school using wearable sensors. *Sensors*, 20(18), 2020.

[517] Inc. The MathWorks. Matlab release 2018b (https://la.mathworks.com/help/matlab/). Available at https://la.mathworks.com/help/matlab/ (accessed: 2021-05-11), 2018.

[518] Thomas Thesen, Carrie R McDonald, Chad Carlson, Werner Doyle, Syd Cash et al. Sequential then interactive processing of letters and words in the left fusiform gyrus. *Nature Communications*, 3(1): 1–8, 2012.

[519] BL Thomas and M Viljoen. Heart rate variability and academic performance of first-year university students. *Neuropsychobiology*, 78(4): 175–181, 2019.

[520] Rhys H Thomas and Samuel F Berkovic. The hidden genetics of epilepsy—A clinically important new paradigm. *Nature Reviews Neurology*, 10(5): 283, 2014.

[521] RS Thorpe. Biometric analysis of geographic variation and racial affinities. *Biological Reviews*, 51(4): 407–452, 1976.

[522] Esteban Tlelo-Cuautle, VH Carbajal-Gomez, PJ Obeso-Rodelo, JJ Rangel-Magdaleno and Jose Cruz Nunez-Perez. Fpga realization of a chaotic communication system applied to image processing. *Nonlinear Dynamics*, 82(4): 1879–1892, 2015.

[523] Esteban Tlelo-Cuautle, L De la Fraga and J Rangel-Magdaleno. *Engineering Applications of FPGAs*. Springer, 2016.

[524] Fernando Torres. Atlas and classification of electroencephalography. *Pediatric Neurology*, 22(4): 332, 2000.

[525] Gema Torres-Luque, Ángel Iván Fernández-García, David Cabello-Manrique, José María Giménez-Egido and Enrique Ortega-Toro. Design and validation of an observational instrument for the technical-tactical actions in singles tennis. *Frontiers in Psychology*, 9: 2418, 2018.

[526] Daisuke Tsuzuki, Hama Watanabe, Ippeita Dan and Gentaro Taga. Minr 10/20 system: Quantitative and reproducible cranial landmark setting method for MRI based on minimum initial reference points. Journal of Neuroscience Methods, 264: 86–93, 2016.

[527] Turker Tuncer, Erhan Akbal and Sengul Dogan. Multileveled ternary pattern and iterative relieff based bird sound classification. *Applied Acoustics*, 176: 107866, 2021.

[528] MA Turk and AP Pentland. Face recognition using eigenfaces. In *Proceedings 1991 IEEE Computer Society Conference on Computer Vision and Pattern Recognition*, pp. 586–591, June 1991.

[529] National Health Service UK. Electroencephalogram (EEG). Available at https://www.nhs.uk/conditions/electroencephalogram/ (Accessed: 2021-05-11), October 2017.

[530] JA Unar, Woo Chaw Seng and Almas Abbasi. A review of biometric technology along with trends and prospects. *Pattern Recognition*, 47(8): 2673–2688, 2014.

[531] Florina Ungureanu, Robert Gabriel Lupu, Adrian Cadar and Adrian Prodan. Neuromarketing and visual attention study using eye tracking techniques. In *2017 21st International Conference on System Theory, Control and Computing (ICSTCC)*, pp. 553–557, 2017.

[532] Mojtaba Valinejadshoubi and Azin Shakibabarough. Ergonomics principles and utilizing it as a remedy for probable work related injuries in construction projects. *International Journal of Advances in Engineering & Technology©IJAET*, 6: 232–245, 2013.

[533] Egon L Van Den Broek. Beyond biometrics. *Procedia Computer Science*, 1(1): 2511–2519, 2010.

[534] Erik van der Spek, Stefan Göbel, Ellen Yi-Luen Do, Esteban Clua and Jannicke Baalsrud Hauge (eds.). *Entertainment Computing and Serious Games: First IFIP TC 14 Joint International Conference, ICEC-JCSG 2019, Arequipa, Peru, November 11–15, 2019, Proceedings*, volume 11863 of *Lecture Notes in Computer Science*. Springer International Publishing, Cham, 2019.

[535] Patrick van Esch, J Stewart Black, Drew Franklin and Mark Harder. Alenabled biometrics in recruiting: Insights from marketers for managers. *Australasian Marketing Journal*, 0(0): j.ausmj.2020.04.003, 0.

[536] Anouk van Westrhenen, Thomas De Cooman, Richard HC Lazeron, Sabine Van Huffel and Roland D Thijs. Ictal autonomic changes as a tool for seizure detection: A systematic review. *Clinical Autonomic Research*, 29(2): 161–181, 2019.

[537] Kaat Vandecasteele, Thomas De Cooman, Ying Gu, Evy Cleeren, Kasper Claes et al. Automated epileptic seizure detection based on wearable ecg and ppg in a hospital environment. *Sensors*, 17(10): 2338, 2017.

[538] Neetu Verma, Teenu Xavier and Deepak Agrawal. Biometric attendance and big data analysis for optimizing work processes. *Studies in Health Technology and Informatics*, 225: 68–72, 2016.

[539] Claudia Gonzalez Viejo, Sigfredo Fuentes, Kate Howell, Damir D Torrico and Frank R Dunshea. Integration of non-invasive biometrics with sensory analysis techniques to assess acceptability of beer by consumers. *Physiology & Behavior*, 200: 139–147, 2019.

[540] Idalis Villanueva, Brett D Campbell, Adam C Raikes, Suzanne H Jones and LeAnn G Putney. A multimodal exploration of engineering students' emotions and electrodermal activity in design activities. *Journal of Engineering Education*, 107(3): 414–441, 2018.

[541] C Ye Vincent, Alireza Mansouri, Nebras M Warsi and George M Ibrahim. Atonic seizures in children: A meta-analysis comparing corpus callosotomy to vagus nerve stimulation. *Child's Nervous System*, 1–9, 2020.

[542] S Von Spiczak, A Caliebe, H Muhle, I Helbig and U Stephani. Genetic causes of epileptic encephalopathies. *Magazine for Epileptology*, 24(2): 108, 2011.

[543] Carballo-Hernández W. *Implementación de un clasificador automático de señales epilépticas de EEG usando descriptores caóticos basado en SVM con un procesador embebido Xilinx Zynq-7000 APSoC*. PhD thesis, Tecnologico de Monterrey, campus Puebla, 2015.

[544] W Li, X Hu, R Gravina and G Fortino. A neuro-fuzzy fatigue-tracking and classification system for wheelchair users. *IEEE Access*, 5: 19420–19431, 2017.

[545] H Wakaumi, K Nakamura and T Matsumura. Development of an automated wheelchair guided by a magnetic ferrite marker lane. *Journal of Rehabilitation Research and Development*, 29(1): 27–34, 1992. Place: United States.

[546] Jun Wang, Jamie Barstein, Lauren E Ethridge, Matthew W Mosconi, Yukari Takarae et al. Resting state eeg abnormalities in autism spectrum disorders. *Journal of Neurodevelopmental Disorders*, 5(1): 1–14, 2013.

[547] Mo Wang, Xin'an Wang, Zhuochen Fan, Fei Chen, Sixu Zhang et al. Research on feature extraction algorithm for plantar pressure image and gait analysis in stroke patients. *Journal of Visual Communication and Image Representation*, 58: 525–531, 2019.

[548] Yuanfa Wang, Zunchao Li, Lichen Feng, Chuang Zheng, Yunhe Guan et al. Hardware architecture of lifting-based discrete wavelet transform and sample entropy for epileptic seizure detection. In *2016 13th IEEE*

International Conference on Solid-State and Integrated Circuit Technology (ICSICT), pp. 1582–1584. IEEE, 2016.

[549] Ze Wang, Yin Li, Anna Rose Childress and John A Detre. Brain entropy mapping using fmri. *PloS One*, 9(3): e89948, 2014.

[550] Edmund Wascher, Holger Heppner and Sven Hoffmann. Towards the measurement of event-related eeg activity in real-life working environments. *International Journal of Psychophysiology*, 91(1): 3–9, 2014.

[551] James W Wheless and Raman Sankar. Treatment strategies for myoclonic seizures and epilepsy syndromes with myoclonic seizures. *Epilepsia*, 44: 27–37, 2003.

[552] Halbert White. *Artificial Neural Networks: Approximation and Learning Theory*. Blackwell Publishers, Inc., 1992.

[553] Kimberley Whitehead, Nick Kane, Alistair Wardrope, Ros Kandler and Markus Reuber. Proposal for best practice in the use of video-eeg when psychogenic non-epileptic seizures are a possible diagnosis. *Clinical Neurophysiology Practice*, 2: 130–139, 2017.

[554] WHO. *WHO Model List of Essential Medicines for Children. 18th List.* Geneive, Switzerland, 2013.

[555] WHO. *WHO Model List of Essential Medicines for Children. 4th List.* Geneive, Switzerland, 2013.

[556] Fokko Pieter Wieringa, Natascha Juliana Hendrika Broers, Jeroen Peter Kooman, Frank M Van Der Sande and Chris Van Hoof. Wearable sensors: Can they benefit patients with chronic kidney disease? *Expert Review of Medical Devices*, 14(7): 505–519, 2017.

[557] Frank H Wilhelm and Paul Grossman. Emotions beyond the laboratory: Theoretical fundaments, study design, and analytic strategies for advanced ambulatory assessment. *Biological Psychology*, 84(3): 552–569, 2010.

[558] Jennifer A Williams, Fodé Abass Cisse, Mike Schaekermann, Foksouna Sakadi, Nana Rahamatou Tassiou et al. Smartphone eeg and remote online interpretation for children with epilepsy in the republic of guinea: Quality, characteristics, and practice implications. *Seizure*, 71: 93–99, 2019.

[559] JoM Wilmshurst, Anne T Berg, Lieven Lagae, Charles R Newton and J Helen Cross. The challenges and innovations for therapy in children with epilepsy. *Nature Reviews Neurology*, 10(5): 249–260, 2014.

[560] Khin Nandar Win, Kenli Li, Jianguo Chen, Philippe Fournier Viger and Keqin Li. Fingerprint classification and identification algorithms for criminal investigation: A survey. *Future Generation Computer Systems*, 110: 758–771, 2020.

[561] M Winterhalder, T Maiwald, HU Voss, R Aschenbrenner-Scheibe, J Timmer and A Schulze-Bonhage. The seizure prediction characteristic: A general framework to assess and compare seizure prediction methods. *Epilepsy & Behavior*, 4(3): 318–325, 2003.

[562] Richard JS Wise, Joshua Greene, Christian Büchel and Sophie K Scott. Brain regions involved in articulation. *The Lancet*, 353(9158): 1057–1061, 1999.

[563] Jonathan R Wolpaw, Niels Birbaumer, Dennis J McFarland, Gert Pfurtscheller and Theresa M Vaughan. Brain–computer interfaces for communication and control. *Clinical Neurophysiology*, 113(6): 767–791, 2002.

[564] Matthew To Worsey, Hugo G Espinosa, Jonathan B Shepherd and David V Thiel. Inertial sensors for performance analysis in combat sports: A systematic review. *Sports (Basel, Switzerland)*, 7(1), Jan 2019.

[565] Bian Wu. An eye tracking study of high- and low-performing students in solving interactive and analytical problems. *Educational Technology & Society*, 20: 10 2017.

[566] Shuen-De Wu, Chiu-Wen Wu, Shiou-Gwo Lin, Chun-Chieh Wang and Kung-Yen Lee. Time series analysis using composite multiscale entropy. *Entropy*, 15(3): 1069–1084, 2013.

[567] Xilinx. ZC702 *Evaluation Board for the Zynq-7000 XC7Z020 All Programmable SoC:User's Guide*. Xilinx, 1.3 edition, 2014.

[568] Lingyu Xu, Yanrong Guo, Jun Li, Jie Yu and Huan Xu. Classification of autism spectrum disorder based on fluctuation entropy of spontaneous hemodynamic fluctuations. *Biomedical Signal Processing and Control*, 60: 101958, 2020.

[569] Rui Xu and Don Wunsch. *Clustering*, volume 10. John Wiley & Sons, 2008.

[570] Shuai Xu, Alina Rwei, Bellington Vwalika, Maureen Chisembele, Jeffrey Stringer et al. Wireless skin sensors for physiological monitoring of infants in low-income and middle-income countries. *The Lancet Digital Health*, 3, 02 2021.

[571] Wenkai Xu and Eung-Joo Lee. Face recognition using wavelets transform and 2d pca by svm classifier. *International Journal of Multimedia and Ubiquitous Engineering*, 9(3): 281–290, 2014.

[572] Drishti Yadav, Shilpee Yadav and Karan Veer. A comprehensive assessment of brain computer interfaces: Recent trends and challenges. *Journal of Neuroscience Methods*, 108918, 2020.

[573] Mahendra Yadava, Pradeep Kumar, Rajkumar Saini, Partha Pratim Roy and Debi Prosad Dogra. Analysis of eeg signals and its application to neuromarketing. *Multimedia Tools and Applications*, 76(18): 19087–19111, Sep 2017.

[574] Roman V Yampolskiy and Venu Govindaraju. Taxonomy of behavioural biometrics. *Behavioral Biometrics for Human Identification: Intelligent Applications*, page 1, 2009.

[575] Jun Yan, Benyu Zhang, Shuicheng Yan, Qiang Yang, Hua Li et al. Immc: Incremental maximum margin criterion. In *Proceedings of the Tenth ACM SIGKDD International Conference on Knowledge Discovery and Data Mining*, KDD'04, pp. 725–730, New York, NY, USA, 2004. Association for Computing Machinery.

[576] Kuo Hui Yeh. A secure IoT-based healthcare system with body sensor networks. *IEEE Access*, 4: 10288–10299, 2016.

[577] Ricardo Zavala Yoe. *Modelling and Control of Dynamical Systems: Numerical Implementation in a Behavioral Framework*, volume 124. Springer, 2008.

[578] Zhiwen Yu, He Du, Dong Xiao, Zhu Wang, Qi Han et al. Recognition of human computer operations based on keystroke sensing by smartphone microphone. *IEEE Internet of Things Journal*, 5(2): 1156–1168, 2018.

[579] Morteza Zabihi, Serkan Kiranyaz, Turker Ince and Moncef Gabbouj. Patient specific epileptic seizure detection in long-term eeg recording in paediatric patients with intractable seizures. In *IET Intelligent Signal Processing Conference 2013 (ISP 2013)*. IET, 2013.

[580] LA Zadeh. Fuzzy sets. *Information and Control*, 8(3): 338–353, June 1965.

[581] Andleeb Zahra, Bilal Hussain, Amer Jamil, Z Ahmed and Shahid Mahboob. Forensic str profiling based smart barcode, a highly efficient and cost effective human identification system. *Saudi Journal of Biological Sciences*, 25(8): 1720–1723, 2018.

[582] Roberto Zangróniz, Arturo Martínez-Rodrigo, José Manuel Pastor, María T López and Antonio Fernández-Caballero. Electrodermal activity sensor for classification of calm/distress condition. *Sensors*, 17(10): 2324, 2017.

[583] Zavala-Yoé Ricardo and Ramírez-Mendoza. Dynamische entropietrajektorien zum gleichzeitigen vergleich von patienten mit doose und lennoxgastaut syndrome. *Zeitschrift für Epileptologie, Springer Medizin*, 32, 2019.

[584] R Zavala-Yoé, R Ramirez-Mendoza and LC Jimenez-Botello. Mathematical complexity as alternative to deal with multiple massive data eegin children epilepsy. *Zeitschrift fuer Epileptologie*, 28(1): 12, 2015.

[585] Ricardo Zavala-Yoé, Ricardo Ramírez-Mendoza and Luz M Cordero. Novel way to investigate evolution of children refractory epilepsy by complexity metrics in massive information. *SpringerPlus*, 4(1): 1–33, 2015.

[586] Ricardo Zavala-Yoe and Ricardo A Ramirez-Mendoza. Dynamic complexity measures and entropy paths for modelling and comparison of evolution of patients with drug resistant epileptic encephalopathy syndromes (drees). *Metabolic Brain Disease*, 32(5): 1553–1569, 2017.

[587] Ricardo Zavala-Yoe, Ricardo A Ramirez-Mendoza and Luz M Cordero. Entropy measures to study and model long term simultaneous evolution of children in doose and lennox–gastaut syndromes. *Journal of Integrative Neuroscience*, 15(02): 205–221, 2016.

[588] Ricardo Zavala-Yoé, Ricardo A Ramírez-Mendoza and Ruben Morales-Menendez. Real time acquisition and processing of massive electroencephalographic signals for modeling by nonlinear statistics. *International Journal on Interactive Design and Manufacturing (IJIDeM)*, 11(2): 427–433, 2017.

[589] Wenbing Zhao, Roanna Lun, Connor Gordon, Abou-Bakar M Fofana, Deborah D Espy et al. A human-centered activity tracking system: Toward a healthier workplace. *IEEE Transactions on Human-Machine Systems*, 47(3): 343–355, 2017.

[590] Hui Zhi and Sanyang Liu. Face recognition based on genetic algorithm. *Journal of Visual Communication and Image Representation*, 58: 495–502, 2019.

[591] Jianguang Zhong, Aizhu Tao, Zhe Xu, Hong Jiang, Yilei Shao et al. Whole eye axial biometry during accommodation using ultra-long scan depth

optical coherence tomography. *American Journal of Ophthalmology*, 157(5): 1064–1069.e2, 2014.

[592] Jia Zhou and Gavriel Salvendy. *Human Aspects of IT for the Aged Population Part 2*. Springer, 2016.

[593] Ruishi Zhou, Chenshuo Wang, Pengfei Zhang, Xianxiang Chen, Lidong Du et al. Ecg-based biometric under different psychological stress states. *Computer Methods and Programs in Biomedicine*, 202: 106005, 2021.

[594] Guohun Zhu, Yan Li, Peng Paul Wen, Shuaifang Wang and Ning Zhong. Unsupervised classification of epileptic eeg signals with multi scale k-means algorithm. In *International Conference on Brain and Health Informatics*, pp. 158–167. Springer, 2013.

[595] Alejandro Enrique Flores Zuniga, Khin Than Win and Willy Susilo. Biometrics for electronic health records. *Journal of Medical Systems*, 34(5): 975–983, 2010.

Index

For Product Safety Concerns and Information please contact our EU
representative GPSR@taylorandfrancis.com
Taylor & Francis Verlag GmbH, Kaufingerstraße 24, 80331 München, Germany